Medical Pharmacology at a Glance

CHRIS NUTT
FACULTY OF MEDICINE (+DENTISTRY)
MBChB - 2nd MB.
UNIVERSITY OF DUNDEE.
1993/1994.

Medical Pharmacology at a Glance

M.J. NEAL
Professor of Pharmacology,
United Medical and Dental Schools of
Guy's and St Thomas's Hospitals (UMDS)
St Thomas's Hospital, Lambeth Palace Road,
London SE1 7EH

SECOND EDITION

OXFORD
BLACKWELL SCIENTIFIC PUBLICATIONS
LONDON EDINBURGH BOSTON
MELBOURNE PARIS BERLIN VIENNA

Editorial Offices:
Osney Mead, Oxford OX2 0EL
25 John Street, London WC1N 2BL
23 Ainslie Place, Edinburgh EH3 6AJ
238 Main Street, Cambridge
Massachusetts 02142, USA
54 University Street, Carlton
Victoria 3053, Australia

Other Editorial Offices:
Librairie Arnette SA
2, rue Casimir-Delavigne
75006 Paris
France

Blackwell Wissenschafts-Verlag GmbH
Meinekestrasse 4
D-1000 Berlin 15
Germany

Blackwell MZV
Feldgasse 13
A-1238 Wien
Austria

First published 1987
Reprinted 1988, 1989 (twice), 1990, 1991 (twice)
Four Dragons edition 1989
Reprinted 1991
Second edition 1992
Reprinted 1993 (twice)
Four Dragons edition 1992
Reprinted 1993 (twice)

Set by Semantic Graphics, Singapore
Printed and bound in Great Britain
by the University Press, Cambridge

DISTRIBUTORS

Marston Book Services Ltd
PO Box 87
Oxford OX2 0DT
(*Orders*: Tel: 0865 791155
Fax: 0865 791927
Telex: 837515)

USA
Blackwell Scientific Publications, Inc.
238 Main Street
Cambridge, MA 02142
(*Orders*: Tel: 800 759–6102
617 876–7000)

Canada
Times Mirror Professional Publishing, Ltd
5240 Finch Avenue East
Scarborough, Ontario M1S 5A2
(*Orders*: Tel: 800 268–4178
416 298–1588)

Australia
Blackwell Scientific Publications Pty Ltd
54 University Street
Carlton, Victoria 3053
(*Orders*: Tel: 03 347–5552)

A catalogue record for this book is available from the British Library

ISBN 0–632–03373–8
ISBN 0–632–03424–6 (Four Dragons)

Contents

Preface

This book is written primarily for preclinical medical students but it should also be useful to students and scientists in other disciplines who would like an elementary and concise introduction to pharmacology.

In this book the text has been reduced to a minimum for understanding the figures. Nevertheless, I have attempted in each chapter to explain how the drugs produce their effects and to outline their uses.

In this second edition most chapters have been updated and some have been completely rewritten. I am most grateful to the readers who have written appreciative letters and to the academics and students who have made helpful suggestions. As a result of these comments I have added chapters on chemotherapy and drug dependence. Some of the diagrams were thought to be over-complicated and I have redrawn them in an effort to make them more readily understood. Any failures in this respect are entirely my responsibilty.

Acknowledgements

I am grateful to Professor J. Ritter, Professor I. Phillips, Professor S.E. File, Dr A.M. Gurney, Dr S.J. Paterson and Dr P.J. Ciclitira who kindly read chapters relating to their special interest and who offered valuable advice and criticism. I am especially grateful to Miss Jean Plaskett for preparing the manuscript.

How to use this book

Each of the chapters (listed on page 5) represents a particular topic, corresponding roughly to a 60-minute lecture. Beginners in pharmacology should start at Chapter 1 and first read through the text on the left-hand pages (which occasionally continues to the facing right-hand page above the ruled line) of several chapters using the figures only as a guide.

Once the general outline has been grasped, it is probably better to concentrate on the *figures* one at a time. Some are quite complicated and can certainly not be taken in 'at a glance'. Each should be studied carefully and worked through together with the *legends* (right-hand pages). Since many drugs appear in more than one chapter, considerable cross-referencing has been provided. As progress is made through the book, use of this cross-referencing will provide valuable reinforcement and a greater understanding of drug action. Once the information has been understood the figures should subsequently require little more than a brief look to refresh the memory.

The figures are highly diagrammatic and not to scale.

Further reading

British National Formulary. British Medical Association and The Pharmaceutical Society of Great Britain, London (about 550 pp). The *BNF* is updated twice a year.

Rang, H.P. & Dale, M.M. (1991) *Pharmacology*, 2nd edn. Churchill Livingstone, Edinburgh (955 pp).

Gilman, A.G., Rall, T.W., Nies, A.S. & Taylor, P. (1990) *The Pharmacological Basis of Therapeutics*, 8th edn. Pergamon Press, Oxford (1811 pp).

1 Introduction: principles of drug action

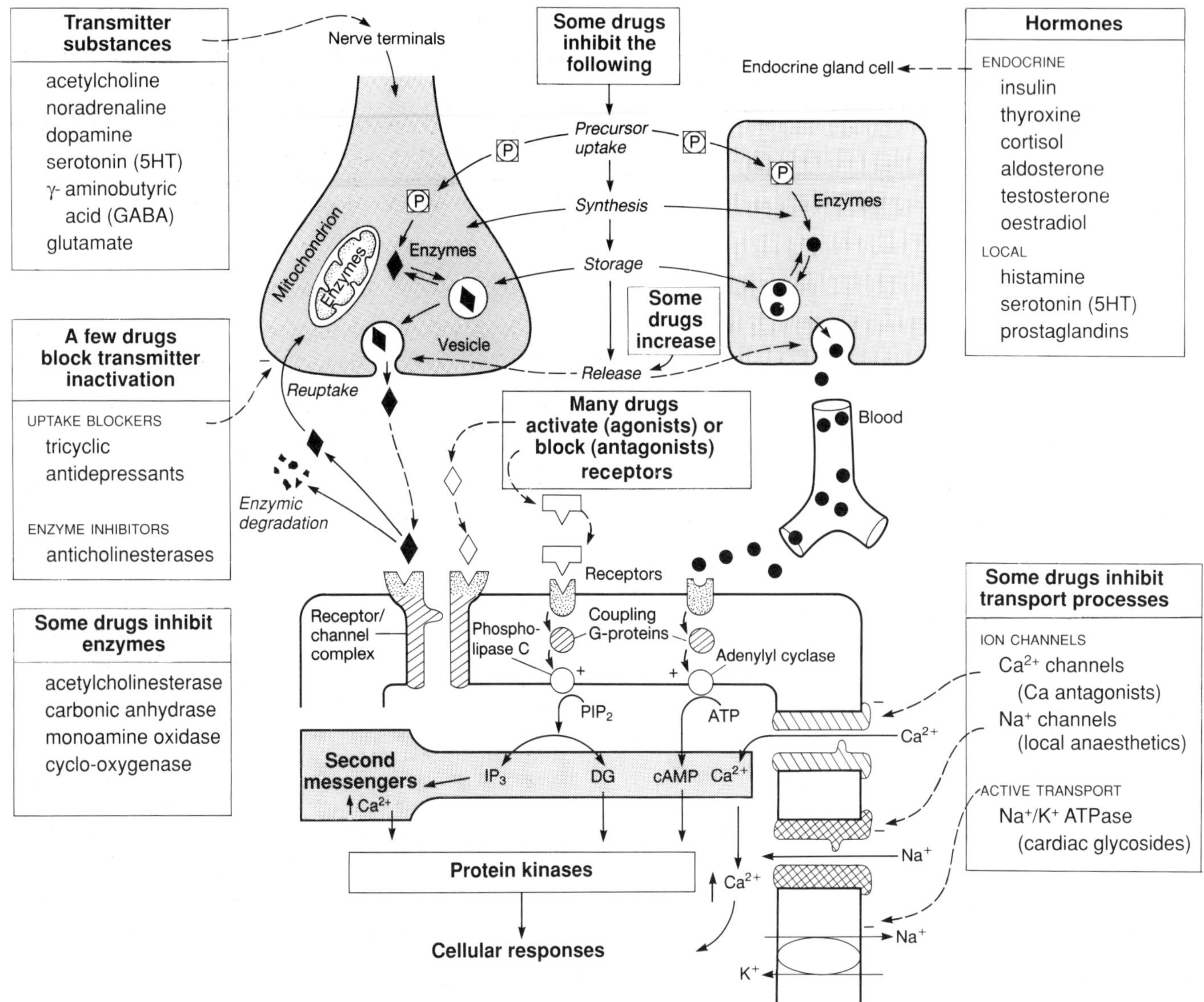

Medical pharmacology is the science of chemicals (drugs) that interact with the human body. These interactions are divided into two classes: **pharmacodynamics**, the effects of the drug on the body, and **pharmacokinetics**, the way the body affects the drug with time (i.e. absorption, distribution, metabolism and excretion).

The most common ways in which a drug can produce its effects are shown in the figure. A few drugs (e.g. general anaesthetics, osmotic diuretics) act by virtue of their physicochemical properties and this is called **non-specific** drug action. Some drugs act as false substrates or inhibitors for certain **transport systems** (bottom right) or **enzymes** (bottom left). Most drugs, however, produce their effects by acting on specific protein molecules, usually located in the cell membrane. These proteins are called **receptors** ( ) and they normally respond to endogenous chemicals in the body. These chemicals are either synaptic **transmitter substances** (top left, ♦) or **hormones** (top right, ●). For example, acetylcholine is a transmitter substance released from motor nerve endings and it activates receptors in skeletal muscle initiating a sequence of events that results in contraction of the muscle. Chemicals (e.g. acetylcholine) or drugs that activate receptors and produce a response are called **agonists**. Some drugs, called **antagonists** ( ), combine with receptors, but do not activate them. Antagonists reduce the probability of the transmitter substance (or another agonist) combining with the receptor and so reduce or block its action.

The activation of receptors by an agonist or hormone is coupled to the physiological or biochemical responses by transduction mechanisms (lower figure) that often (but not always) involve molecules called **'second messengers'** ( ).

The interaction between a drug and the binding site of the receptor depends on the complementarity of 'fit' of the two molecules. The closer the fit and the greater the number of bonds (usually non-covalent), the stronger will be the attractive forces between them, and the higher the **affinity** of the drug for the receptor. The ability of a drug to combine with one particular type of receptor is called **specificity**. No drug is truly specific but many have a relatively **selective** action on one type of receptor.

Drugs are prescribed to produce a therapeutic effect but they often produce additional **unwanted effects** which range from the trivial (e.g. slight nausea) to the fatal (e.g. aplastic anaemia).

RECEPTORS

These are protein molecules which are normally activated by transmitters or hormones. Many receptors have now been cloned and their amino acid sequences determined. Agonist gated receptors are made up from subunits which form a central ion channel (e.g. nicotinic receptor, Chapter 6). G-protein-coupled-receptors (see below) form a family of receptors with seven membrane-spanning helices.

Transmitter substances are chemicals released from nerve terminals which diffuse across the synaptic cleft and bind to the receptors. This activates the receptors, presumably by changing their conformation, and triggers a sequence of post-synaptic events resulting in, for example, muscle contraction or glandular secretion. Following its release, the transmitter is inactivated (left of figure) by either enzymic degradation (e.g. acetylcholine) or reuptake (e.g. noradrenaline, γ-aminobutyric acid). Many drugs act by either reducing or enhancing synaptic transmission.

Hormones are chemicals released into the bloodstream; they produce their physiological effects on tissues possessing the necessary specific hormone receptors. Drugs may interact with the endocrine system by inhibiting (e.g. antithyroid drugs, Chapter 33) or increasing (e.g. oral antidiabetic agents, Chapter 34) hormone release. Other drugs interact with hormone receptors which may be activated (e.g. steroidal anti-inflammatory drugs, Chapter 31) or blocked (e.g. oestrogen antagonists, Chapter 32). Local hormones (autacoids) such as histamine, serotonin (5-hydroxytryptamine, 5HT), kinins and prostaglandins are released in pathological processes. The effects of histamine can sometimes be blocked with antihistamines (Chapter 11) and drugs that block prostaglandin synthesis (e.g. aspirin) are widely used as anti-inflammatory agents (Chapter 30).

TRANSPORT SYSTEMS

The lipid cell membrane provides a barrier against the transport of hydrophilic molecules into or out of the cell.

Ion channels are selective pores in the membrane that allow the ready transfer of ions down their electrochemical gradient. The open–closed state of these channels is controlled either by the membrane potential (voltage-sensitive channels) or by transmitter substances. Some channels (e.g. Ca^{2+} channels in the heart) are both voltage and transmitter sensitive. Important examples of drugs that act on ionic channels are the *calcium antagonists* (Chapter 16) and *local anaesthetics* (Chapter 5).

Active transport processes are used to transfer substances against their concentration gradients. They utilize special carrier molecules in the membrane and require metabolic energy. Two examples are:

Sodium pump. This expels Na^+ ions from inside the cell by a mechanism that derives energy from adenosine triphosphate (ATP) and involves the enzyme ATPase. The carrier is linked to the transfer of K^+ ions into the cell. The *cardiac glycosides* (Chapter 18) act by inhibiting the Na^+/K^+ ATPase. Na^+ and/or Cl^- transport processes in the kidney are inhibited by some *diuretics* (Chapter 14).

Noradrenaline transport. The *tricyclic antidepressants* (Chapter 27) prolong the action of noradrenaline by blocking its reuptake into central nerve terminals.

ENZYMES

These are catalytic proteins that increase the *rate* of chemical reactions in the body. Drugs that act by inhibiting enzymes include *anticholinesterases* which enhance the action of acetylcholine (Chapters 6 and 8), *carbonic anhydrase inhibitors* which are diuretics (i.e. increase urine flow, Chapter 14), *monoamine oxidase inhibitors* which are antidepressants (Chapter 27) and inhibitors of *cyclo-oxygenase* (e.g. aspirin, Chapter 30).

SECOND MESSENGERS

These are chemicals whose intracellular concentration increases or, more rarely, decreases in response to receptor activation by agonists and trigger processes that eventually result in a cellular response. The most studied second messengers are: Ca^{2+} ions, cyclic adenosine monophosphate (cAMP), inositol-1,4,5-triphosphate (IP_3) and diacylgycerol (DG).

cAMP is formed from ATP by the enzyme adenylyl cyclase when, for example, β-adrenoceptors are stimulated. The cAMP activates an enzyme (protein kinase A) which phosphorylates a protein (enzyme or ion channel) leading to a physiological effect.

IP_3 and DG are formed from membrane phosphatidylinositol 4,5-biphosphate by activation of a phospholipase C. Both messengers can, like cAMP, activate kinases, but IP_3 does this indirectly by mobilizing intracellular calcium stores. Some muscarinic effects of acetylcholine and α_1-adrenergic effects involve this mechanism (Chapter 7).

G-proteins. The stimulation of adenylyl cyclase and phosphokinase C following receptor activation is mediated by a family of regulatory guanosine triphosphate (GTP)-binding proteins (G-proteins). The receptor–agonist complex induces a conformational change in the G-protein, causing its α-subunit to bind GTP. α-GTP dissociates from the G-protein and activates (or inhibits) the enzyme. The signal to the enzyme ends because α-GTP has intrinsic GTPase activity and turns itself off by hydrolysing the GTP to GDP. α-GDP then reassociates with the βγ G-protein subunits.

UNWANTED DRUG EFFECTS

Adverse effects related to dosage. A drug that acts on a receptor type which is present in many tissues will cause predictable adverse effects. For example, *atropine* blocks acetylcholine receptors which are present in the viscera, eye, skin and brain, and whatever the drug is given for, it is likely to cause blurred vision, dry mouth, constipation and urinary retention (Chapter 8). Some drugs act on several different types of receptors. For example, the beneficial effects of *chlorpromazine* in schizophrenia result from blocking dopamine receptors in the brain, but the drug also blocks acetylcholine receptors and may produce the effects described for atropine. Many unwanted effects are simply due to extension of the drug's action. Thus, overdosage of the anticoagulant, *heparin*, causes bleeding.

Adverse effects not related to dosage. These include *hypersensitivity reactions*, which are harmful immunological responses to drugs.

2 Drug–receptor interactions

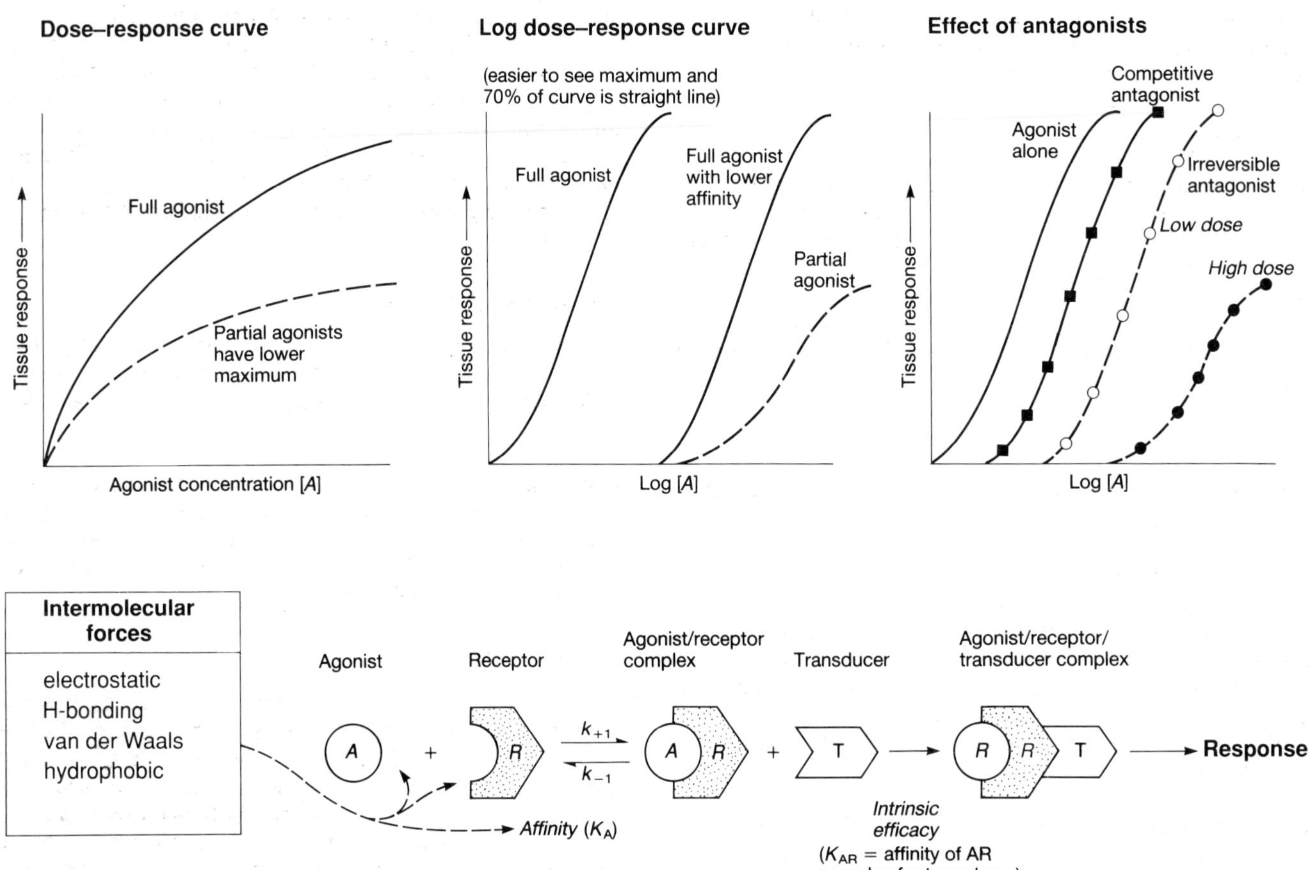

The tissues in the body have only a few basic responses when exposed to agonists (e.g. muscle contraction, glandular secretion) and the quantitative relationship between these physiological responses and the concentration of the agonist can be measured by using **bioassays**. The first part of the drug–receptor interaction, i.e. the binding of drug to receptor, can be studied in isolation using **binding assays**.

It has been found by experiment that for many tissues and agonists, when the response is plotted against the concentration of the drug, a curve is produced that is often hyperbolic (**dose–response curve**, top left). In practice, it is often more convenient to plot the response against the logarithm of the agonist concentration (**log dose–response curve**, middle top). Assuming the interaction between the drug (A) and the receptor (R) (lower figure) obeys the law of mass action, then the concentration of drug–receptor complex (AR) is given by:

$$[AR] = \frac{[R_O][A]}{K_D + [A]}$$

where R_o = total concentration of receptors, A = agonist concentration, K_D = dissociation constant, and AR = concentration of occupied receptors.

Since this is the equation for a hyperbola, the shape of the dose–response curve is explained if the response is directly proportional to $[AR]$. Unfortunately, this simple theory does not explain another experimental finding—some agonists, called **partial agonists**, cannot elicit the same maximum response as full agonists even if they have the same affinity for the receptor (top left and middle, ----). Thus, in addition to having affinity for the receptor, an agonist has another chemical property called **intrinsic efficacy** which is its ability to elicit a response when it binds to a receptor (lower figure).

A **competitive antagonist** has no intrinsic efficacy and effectively dilutes the receptor concentration. This causes a parallel shift of the log dose–response curve to the right (top right, ■) but the maximum response is not depressed. In contrast, **irreversible antagonists** depress the maximum response (top right, ●). However, at low concentrations a parallel shift of the log dose–response curve may occur without a reduction in the maximum response (top right, ○). Since an irreversible antagonist in effect removes receptors from the system, it is clear that not all the receptors need to be occupied to elicit the maximum response (i.e. there is a **receptor reserve**).

INTERMOLECULAR FORCES

Drug molecules in the environment of receptors are attracted initially by relatively long-range electrostatic forces. Then, if the molecule is suitably shaped to fit closely to the binding site of the receptor, hydrogen bonds and van der Waal forces briefly bind the drug to the receptor. Irreversible antagonists bind to receptors with strong covalent bonds.

AFFINITY

This is a measure of how avidly a drug binds to its receptor. It is characterized by the equilibrium dissociation constant (K_D) which is the ratio of rate constants for the reverse (k_{-1}) and forward (k_{+1}) reaction between the drug and the receptor. The reciprocal of K_D is called the affinity constant (K_A) and (in the absence of receptor reserve, see below) is the concentration of drug that produces 50% of the maximum response.

ANTAGONISTS

These are drugs that bind to receptors but do not activate them. They may be competitive or irreversible.

Competitive antagonists bind reversibly with receptors and the tissue response can be returned to normal by increasing the dose of agonist, because this increases the probability of agonist–receptor collisions at the expense of antagonist–receptor collisions. The ability of higher doses of agonist to overcome the effects of the antagonist results in parallel shift of the dose–response curve to the right and is the hallmark of competitive antagonism.

Irreversible antagonists (e.g. phenoxybenzamine) have an effect which cannot be reversed by increasing the concentration of agonist.

RECEPTOR RESERVE

In many tissues, irreversible antagonists initially shift the log dose–response curve to the right without reducing the maximum response, indicating that the maximum response can be obtained without the agonist occupying all the receptors. The excess receptors are sometimes called '*spare*' receptors, but this is a misleading term because they are of functional significance. They increase both the sensitivity and speed of a system because the concentration of drug–receptor complex (and hence the response) depends on the product of the agonist concentration and the *total* receptor concentration.

PARTIAL AGONIST

This is an agonist that cannot elicit the same maximum response as a 'full' agonist. The reasons for this are unknown. Recently, it has been suggested that agonism depends on the affinity of the drug–receptor complex for a *transducer molecule* (lower figure). Thus a full agonist produces a complex with high affinity for the transducer (e.g. the coupling G-proteins, Chapter 1) whilst a partial agonist–receptor complex has a lower affinity for the transducer and so cannot elicit the full response.

When acting at receptors alone, partial agonists stimulate a physiological response, but they antagonize the effects of a full agonist (e.g. some β-adrenoceptor antagonists, Chapters 15 and 16).

INTRINSIC EFFICACY

This is the ability of an agonist to alter the conformation of a receptor in such a way that it elicits a response in the system. It is defined as the affinity of the agonist–receptor complex for a transducer.

Partial agonists and receptor reserve. A drug that is a partial agonist in a tissue with no receptor reserve may be a full agonist in a tissue possessing many 'spare' receptors because its poor efficacy can be offset by activating a larger number of receptors than required by a full agonist.

BIOASSAY

These involve the use of a biological tissue to relate drug concentration to a physiological response. Usually, isolated tissues are used because it is then easier to control the drug concentration around the tissue and reflex responses are abolished. Bioassays can be used to estimate: (1) the concentration of a drug; (2) its binding constants; or (3) its potency relative to another drug. Measurement of the relative potencies of a series of agonists on different tissues has been one of the main ways used to classify receptors, e.g. adrenoceptors (Chapter 7).

BINDING ASSAYS

These are simple and very adaptable. Membrane fragments from homogenized tissues are incubated with radiolabelled drug (usually ^3H) and then recovered by filtration. After correction for non-specific binding, the ^3H-drug bound to the receptors can be determined and estimations made of K_A and B_{max} (number of binding sites). Binding assays are widely used to study drug receptors (see for example Chapters 26 and 27) but have the disadvantage that no functional response is measured and often the radiolabelled drug does not bind to a single class of receptor.

3 Drug absorption, distribution and excretion

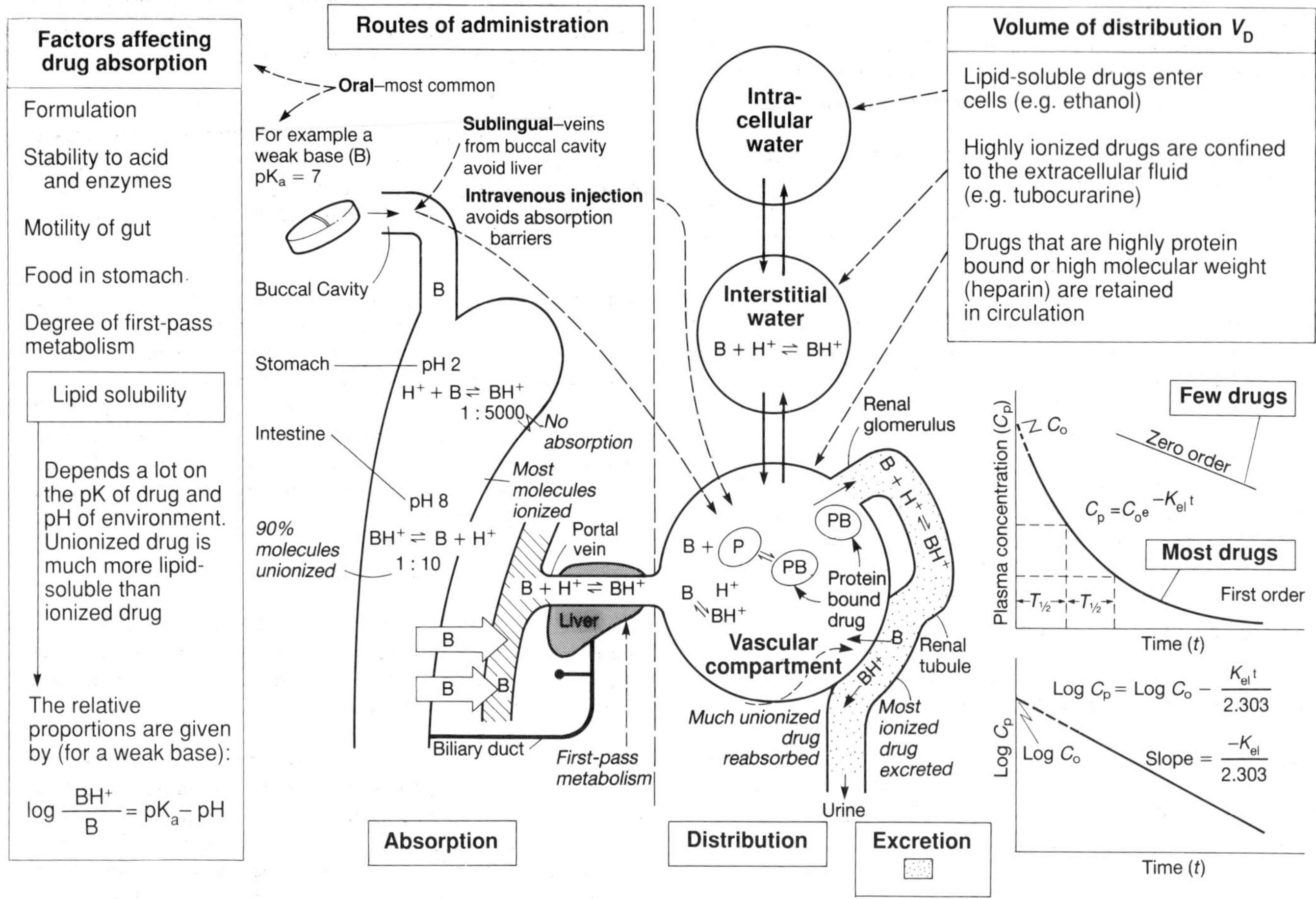

Most drugs are given **orally** and they must pass through the gut wall to enter the bloodstream (left of figure, ⇨). This **absorption** process is affected by many factors (left) but is usually proportional to the **lipid solubility** of the drug. Thus, the absorption of unionized molecules (B) is favoured because they are far more lipid-soluble than those that are ionized (BH^+) and surrounded by a 'shell' of water molecules. Drugs absorbed from the gastrointestinal tract enter the portal circulation (left, ▨) and some are extensively metabolized as they pass through the liver (first-pass metabolism).

Drugs that are sufficiently lipid-soluble to be readily absorbed orally are rapidly distributed throughout the body water compartments (○). Many drugs are loosely bound to plasma albumin, an equilibrium forming between the bound (PB) and free drug (B) in the plasma. Drug that is bound to plasma proteins is confined to the vascular system and is not able to exert its pharmacological actions.

If a drug is given by **intravenous injection**, it enters the blood and is rapidly distributed to the tissues. By taking repeated blood samples, the fall in plasma concentration of the drug with time can be measured (i.e. the rate of drug elimination is measured; right, top graph). Often the concentration falls rapidly at first, but then the rate of decline progressively decreases. Such a curve is called **exponential**, and means that at any given time a **constant fraction** of the drug present is eliminated in unit time. Many drugs show an exponential fall in plasma concentration because the rates at which the drug elimination processes work are themselves usually proportional to the concentration of drug in the plasma. These processes are:

1 Elimination in the urine by glomerular filtration (right, ░).
2 Metabolism, usually by the liver.
3 Uptake by the liver and subsequent elimination in the bile (solid line from liver).

A process that depends on the concentration at any given time is called **first order** and most drugs exhibit first-order elimination kinetics. If any enzyme system responsible for drug metabolism becomes **saturated** then the elimination kinetics change to **zero order**, i.e. the rate of elimination proceeds at a constant rate and is unaffected by an increased concentration of the drug (e.g. ethanol, phenytoin).

ROUTES OF ADMINISTRATION

Drugs can be administered orally or parenterally (i.e. by a non-gastrointestinal route).

Oral. Most drugs are absorbed by this route and because of its convenience it is the most widely used. However, some drugs (e.g. benzylpenicillin, insulin) are destroyed by the acid or enzymes in the gut and must be given parenterally.

Intravenous injection enters the drug directly into the circulation and bypasses the absorption barriers. It is used: (1) where a rapid effect is required; (2) for continuous administration (infusion); (3) for large volumes; and (4) for drugs that cause local tissue damage if given by other routes.

Intramuscular and subcutaneous injections. Drugs in aqueous solution are usually absorbed fairly rapidly, but absorption can be slowed by giving the drug in the form of an ester (e.g. neuroleptic depot preparations, see Chapter 26).

Other routes include *inhalation* (e.g. volatile anaesthetics, some drugs used in asthma), and *topical* (e.g. ointments). *Sublingual* and *rectal* administration avoid the portal circulation, and sublingual preparations in particular, are valuable in giving drugs subject to a high degree of first-pass metabolism.

DISTRIBUTION AND EXCRETION

Distribution around the body occurs when the drug reaches the circulation. It must then penetrate tissues to act.

$t_{\frac{1}{2}}$ (half-life) is the time taken for the concentration of drug in blood to fall by half its original value (right, top graph). Measurement of $t_{\frac{1}{2}}$ allows calculation of the *elimination rate constant* (K_{el}) from the formula:

$$K_{el} = \frac{0.69}{t}$$

K_{el} is the fraction of drug present at any time that would be eliminated in unit time (e.g. $K_{el} = 0.02$ minute^{-1} means that 2% of the drug present is eliminated in 1 minute).

The exponential curve of plasma concentration (C_p) against time (t) is described by:

$$C_p = C_0 e^{-K_{el}t}$$

where C_0 = the initial apparent plasma concentration. By taking logarithms, the exponential curve can be transformed into a more convenient straight line (right, bottom graph) from which C_0 and $t_{\frac{1}{2}}$ can readily be determined.

Volume of distribution (V_D) This is the *apparent* volume into which the drug is distributed. Following an intravenous injection,

$$V_D = \frac{\text{dose}}{C_0}$$

A value of $V_D < 5$ litres implies that the drug is retained within the vascular compartment. A value < 15 litres suggests that the drug is restricted to the extracellular fluid, whilst large volumes of distribution ($V_D > 15$ litres) indicate distribution throughout the total body water or concentration in certain tissues. The volume of distribution can be used to calculate the *clearance* of the drug.

Clearance is an important concept in pharmacokinetics. It is the volume of blood or plasma cleared of drug in unit time. Plasma clearance (Cl_p) is given by the relationship:

$$Cl_p = V_D K_{el}$$

The rate of elimination = $Cl_p \times C_p$. Clearance is the sum of individual clearance values. Thus $Cl_p = Cl_m$ (metabolic clearance) + Cl_r (renal excretion). Clearance, but not $t_{\frac{1}{2}}$, provides an indication of the ability of the liver and kidney to dispose of drugs.

Drug dosage. Clearance values can be used to plan dosage regimens. Ideally in drug treatment, a steady-state plasma concentration ($C_{p\,ss}$) is required within a known therapeutic range. A steady state will be achieved when the rate of drug entering the systemic circulation (dosage rate) equals the rate of elimination. Thus, the dosing rate = $Cl \times C_{p\,ss}$. This equation could be applied to an intravenous infusion because all the dose enters the circulation at a known rate. For oral administration, the equation becomes:

$$\frac{F \times \text{dose}}{\text{dosing interval}} = Cl_p \times C_p\text{, average}$$

where F = *bioavailability* of the drug. The $t_{\frac{1}{2}}$ value of a drug is useful in choosing a dosing interval that does not produce excessively high peaks (toxic levels) and low troughs (ineffective levels) in drug concentration.

Bioavailability is a term used to describe the proportion of administered drug reaching the systemic circulation. Bioavailability is 100% following an intravenous injection ($F = 1$), but drugs are usually given orally and the proportion of the dose reaching the systemic circulation varies with different drugs and also from patient to patient. Drugs subject to a high degree of first-pass metabolism may be almost inactive orally (e.g. glyceryl trinitrate, lignocaine).

EXCRETION

Renal excretion is ultimately responsible for the elimination of most drugs. Drugs appear in the glomerular filtrate, but if they are lipid-soluble they are readily reabsorbed in the renal tubules by passive diffusion. Metabolism of a drug often results in a less lipid-soluble compound, aiding renal excretion (see Chapter 4).

The ionization of weak acids and bases depends on the pH of the tubular fluid. Manipulation of the urine pH is sometimes useful in increasing renal excretion. For example, bicarbonate administration makes the urine alkaline; this ionizes aspirin making it less lipid-soluble and increasing its rate of excretion.

Weak acids and weak bases are actively secreted in the proximal tubule. Penicillins are eliminated by this route.

Biliary excretion. Some drugs (e.g. stilboestrol) are concentrated in the bile and excreted into the intestine where they may be reabsorbed. This entero-hepatic circulation increases the persistence of a drug in the body.

4 Drug metabolism

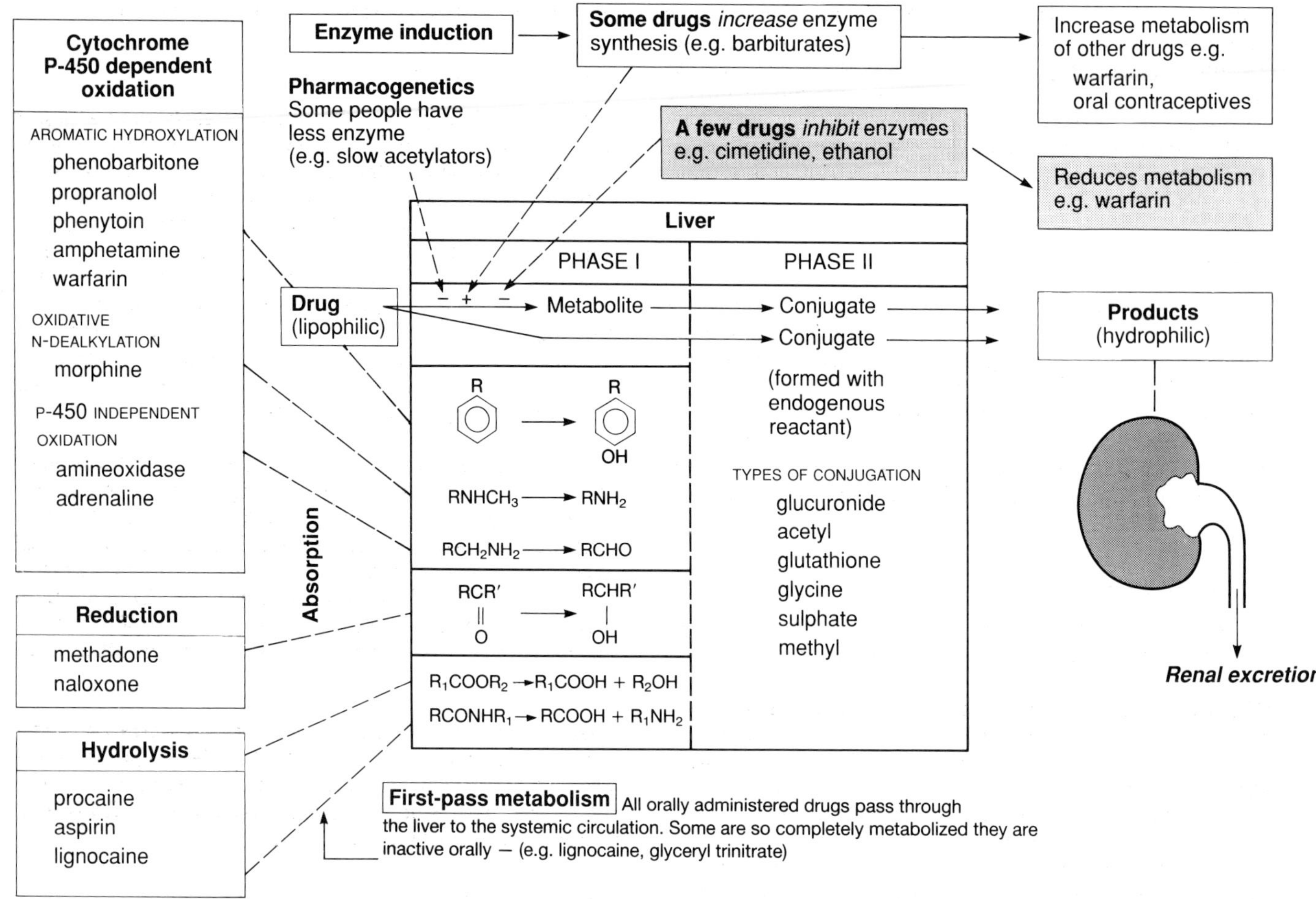

Drug metabolism has two important effects:

1 The drug is made more **hydrophilic**—this hastens its excretion by the kidneys (right, ▩) because the less lipid-soluble metabolite is not readily reabsorbed in the renal tubules.

2 The metabolites are usually **less active** than the parent drug. However, this is not always so, and sometimes the metabolites are as active (or more active) as the original drug. For example, diazepam (a drug use to treat anxiety) is metabolized to nordiazepam and oxazepam, both of which are active. **Prodrugs** are inactive until metabolized in the body to the active drug. For example, levodopa, an anti-parkinsonian drug (Chapter 25), is metabolized to dopamine, whilst the hypotensive drug methyldopa (Chapter 15) is metabolized to α-methylnoradrenaline.

The **liver** is the main organ of drug metabolism and is involved in two general types of reaction:

Phase I reactions involve the biotransformation of a drug to a more polar metabolite (left of figure) by introducing or unmasking a functional group (e.g. -OH, $-NH_2$, -SH).

Oxidations are the most common reactions and these are catalysed by an important class of enzymes called the mixed function oxidases (**cytochrome P-450s**). The substrate specificity of this enzyme complex is very low and many different drugs can be oxidized (examples, top left). Other Phase I reactions are **reductions** (middle left) and **hydrolyses** (bottom left).

Phase II reactions. Drugs or Phase I metabolites that are not sufficiently polar to be excreted rapidly by the kidneys are made more hydrophilic by **conjugation** with endogenous compounds in the liver (centre of figure).

Repeated administration of some drugs (top) increases the synthesis of cytochrome P-450 (**enzyme induction**). This increases the rate of metabolism of the inducing drug and also other drugs metabolized by the same enzyme (top right). In contrast, drugs sometimes **inhibit** microsomal enzyme activity (top, ▩) and this increases the action of drugs metabolized by the same enzyme (top right, □).

In addition to these drug–drug interactions, the metabolism of drugs may be influenced by **genetic factors** (pharmacogenetics), age and some diseases, especially those affecting the liver.

DRUGS

A few drugs (e.g. gallamine, Chapter 6) are highly polar because they are fully ionized at physiological pH. Such drugs are metabolized little, if at all, and the termination of their actions depends mainly on renal excretion. Most drugs, however, are highly lipophilic and are often bound to plasma proteins. Since the protein-bound drug is not filtered at the renal glomerulus and the free drug readily diffuses back from the tubule into the blood, such drugs would have a very prolonged action if their removal relied on renal excretion alone. In general, drugs are metabolized to more polar compounds, which are more easily excreted by the kidneys.

LIVER

The main organ of drug metabolism is the liver, but other organs, such as the gastrointestinal tract and lungs, have considerable activity. Drugs given orally are usually absorbed in the small intestine and enter the portal system to the liver, where they may be extensively metabolized (e.g. lignocaine, morphine, propranolol). This is called *first-pass metabolism*, a term that does not refer only to hepatic metabolism. For example, chlorpromazine is metabolized more in the intestine than by the liver.

PHASE I REACTIONS

The most common reaction is *oxidation*. Other, relatively uncommon, reactions are *reduction* and *hydrolysis*.

Microsomal mixed function oxidase system. Many of the enzymes involved in drug metabolism are located on the smooth endoplasmic reticulum which forms small vesicles when the tissue is homogenized. These vesicles can be isolated by differential centrifugation and are called microsomes.

Microsomal drug oxidations involve NADPH, oxygen and two key enzymes: (1) a flavoprotein, NADPH-cytochrome P-450 reductase; and (2) a haemoprotein, cytochrome P-450, which acts as a terminal oxidase.

Enzyme induction. Some drugs increase cytochrome P-450 activity by either increasing its synthesis or reducing its degradation. Different drugs can induce forms of cytochrome P-450 which have different substrate specificities. For example, phenobarbitone induces cytochrome P-450b, whilst 3-methylcholanthrene (a polycyclic aromatic hydrocarbon) induces cytochrome P-448. The benzo[*a*]pyrene in tobacco smoke will induce cytochrome P-448 and smokers may show increased rates of drug metabolism.

Not all enzymes subject to induction are microsomal. For example, hepatic alcohol dehydrogenase occurs in the cytoplasm.

PHASE II REACTIONS

These usually occur in the liver and involve conjugation of a drug or its Phase I metabolite with an endogenous substance. The resulting conjugates are almost always less active and are polar molecules that are readily excreted by the kidneys.

PHARMACOGENETICS

The study of how genetic determinants affect drug action is called *pharmacogenetics*. The response to drugs varies between individuals and because the variations usually have a Gaussian distribution, it is assumed that the determinant of the response is multifactorial. However, some drug responses show discontinuous variation and in these cases the population can be divided into two or more groups, suggesting a single-gene polymorphism. An important example of polymorphism is debrisoquine hydroxylation. About 5% of the population are poor hydroxylators and show exaggerated and prolonged responses to drugs such as propranolol and metoprolol (Chapter 15), which undergo extensive hepatic metabolism.

Drug-acetylating enzymes. Hepatic *N*-acetylase displays genetic polymorphism. About 50% of the population acetylate isoniazid (an antitubercular drug) rapidly, whilst the other 50% acetylates it slowly. Slow acetylation is due to an autosomal recessive gene which is associated with a smaller amount of hepatic *N*-acetylase. Slow acetylators are more likely to accumulate the drug and to experience adverse reactions. There is evidence for polymorphism in the acetylation of other drugs (e.g. hydralazine).

Plasma pseudocholinesterase. Four separate genes for this enzyme occur at one locus. Rarely ($< 1:2500$) atypical or silent forms of the enzyme occur and these are associated with a grossly prolonged action of suxamethonium, a frequently used neuromuscular blocking drug.

METABOLISM AND DRUG TOXICITY

Occasionally, reactive products of drug metabolism are toxic to various organs, especially the liver. *Paracetamol*, a widely used weak analgesic, normally undergoes glucuronidation and sulphation. However, these processes become saturated at high doses and the drug is then conjugated with glutathione. If the glutathione supply becomes depleted, then a reactive and potentially lethal hepatotoxic metabolite accumulates. Paracetamol is one of the few cases of poisoning where an 'antidote' is available. This is N-*acetylcysteine* which provides -SH groups for the metabolism of the reactive intermediate.

5 Local anaesthetics

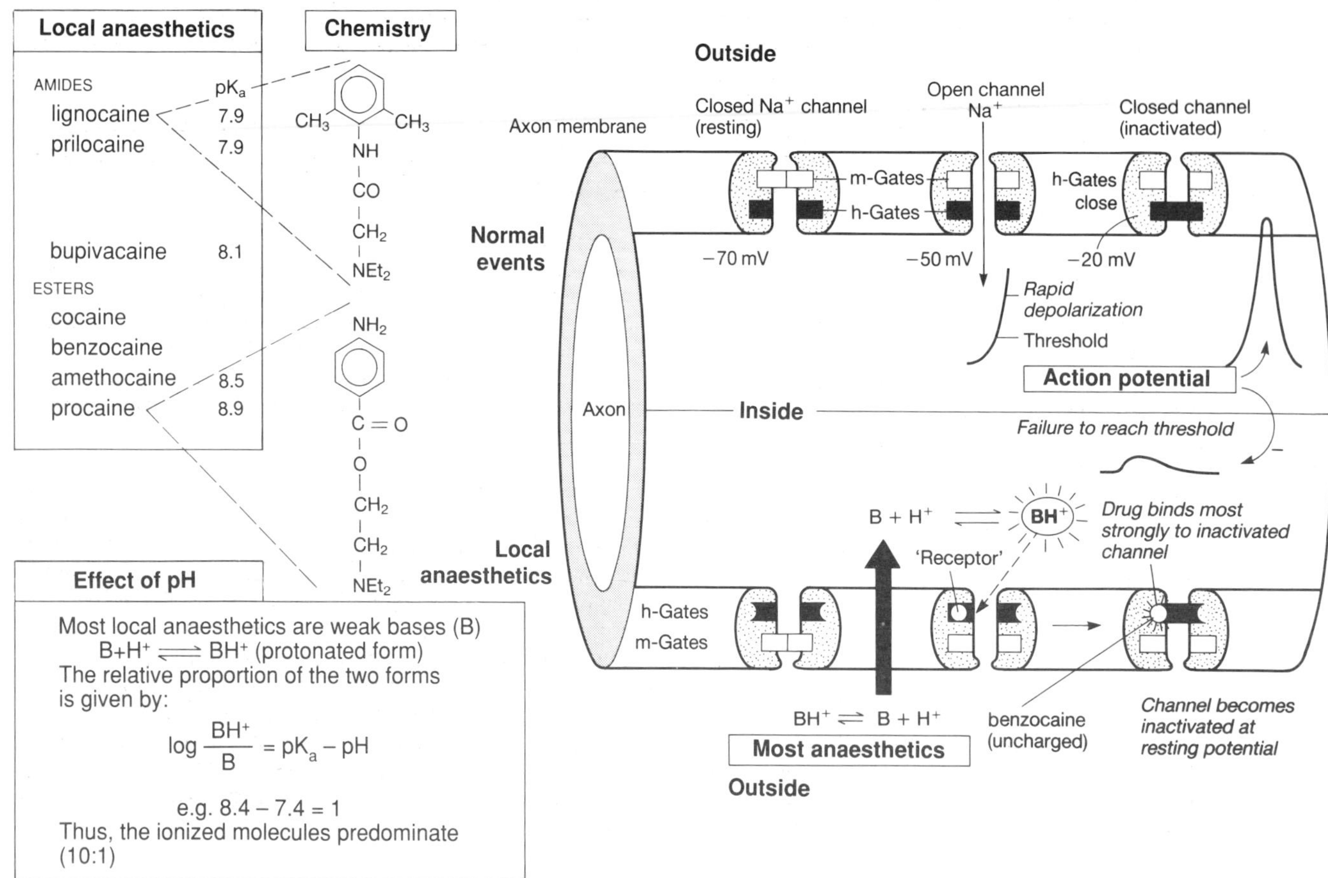

LOCAL ANAESTHETICS

Local anesthetics (top left) are drugs used to prevent pain by causing a reversible block of conduction along nerve fibres. Most are weak bases that exist mainly in a protonated form at body pH (bottom left). The drugs penetrate the nerve in a non-ionized (lipophilic) form (➡), but once inside the axon, some ionized molecules are formed and these block the **Na^+ channels** (▢) preventing the generation of **action potentials** (lower figure).

All nerve fibres are sensitive to local anaesthetics but, in general, small-diameter fibres are more sensitive than large fibres. Thus, a **differential block** can be achieved where the smaller pain and autonomic fibres are blocked, whilst coarse touch and movement are spared. Local anaesthetics vary widely in their potency, duration of action, toxicity and ability to penetrate mucous membranes.

Local anaesthetics depress other excitable tissues (e.g. myocardium) if the concentration in the blood is sufficiently high, but their main systemic effects involve the central nervous system. Synthetic agents produce sedation and light-headedness, although anxiety and restlessness sometimes occur, presumably because central inhibitory synapses are depressed. Higher, toxic doses cause twitching and visual disturbances, whilst severe toxicity causes convulsions and coma, with respiratory and cardiac depression, resulting from medullary depression. Even cocaine, which has central stimulant properties unrelated to its local anaesthetic action, may cause death by respiratory depression.

Lignocaine is the most widely used agent. It acts more rapidly and is more stable than most other local anaesthetics. It has a duration of action of about 90 minutes. *Prilocaine* is similar to lignocaine but is more extensively metabolized and is less toxic in equipotent doses. *Bupivacaine* has a slow onset (up to 30 minutes) but a very long duration of action, up to 8 hours when used for nerve blocks. It is often used in pregnancy to produce continuous epidural blockade during labour. *Benzocaine* is a neutral, water-insoluble, local anaesthetic of low potency. Its only use is in **surface anaesthesia** for non-inflamed tissue (e.g. mouth and pharynx). The more toxic agents, *amethocaine* and *cocaine* have restricted use. Cocaine is primarily used for surface anaesthesia where its intrinsic vasoconstrictor action is desirable (e.g. in the nose). Amethocaine drops are used in ophthalmology to anaesthetize the cornea, but less toxic drugs such as *oxybuprocaine* and *proxymetacaine* which cause much less initial stinging are better.

Hypersensitivity reactions may occur with local anaesthetics, especially in atopic patients, and more often with procaine and other esters of *p*-aminobenzoic acid.

Na^+ CHANNELS

Excitable tissues possess special 'voltage-sensitive' Na^+ channels. Their conductance (gNa^+) is given by $gNa^+ = \bar{g}Na^+ m^3h$ where $\bar{g}Na^+$ is the maximum conductance possible, and m and h are gating constants which depend on the membrane potential. In the figure, these constants are shown schematically as physical gates within the channel. At the resting potential, most h-gates are open and the m-gates are closed (closed channel). Depolarization causes the m-gates to open (open channel) but the intense depolarization of the action potential then causes the h-gates to close the channel (inactivation). This sequence is shown in the upper half of the figure (left to right).

ACTION POTENTIAL

If enough Na^+ channels are opened then the rate of Na^+ entry into the axon exceeds the rate of K^+ exit and at this point, the threshold potential, entry of Na^+ ions further depolarizes the membrane. This opens more Na^+ channels resulting in further depolarization which opens more Na^+ channels and so on. The fast inward Na^+ current quickly depolarizes the membrane towards the Na^+ equilibrium potential (around +67 mV). Then, inactivation of the Na^+ channels and the continuing efflux of K^+ ions causes repolarization of the membrane. Finally, the Na^+ channels regain their normal 'excitable' state and the Na^+ pump restores the lost K^+ and removes the gained Na^+ ions.

MECHANISM OF LOCAL ANAESTHETICS

Local anaesthetics *penetrate* into the interior of the axon in the form of the lipid-soluble free base. There, protonated molecules are formed which then enter and *block* the Na^+ channels after binding to a '*receptor*'. Thus, quaternary (fully protonated) local anaesthetics only work if they are injected inside the nerve axon. Uncharged agents (e.g. benzocaine) dissolve in the membrane and, whilst expansion of the membrane might be expected to compress the Na^+ channels, eventually blocking the passage of Na^+ ions, it seems the channels are blocked in an all-or-none manner. Thus, ionized and non-ionized molecules act in essentially the same way; that is, by binding to a 'receptor' on the Na^+ channel. This 'blocks' the channel largely by preventing the opening of h-gates (i.e. by increasing inactivation). Eventually, so many channels are inactivated that their number falls below the minimum necessary for depolarization to reach threshold, and because action potentials cannot be generated, nerve block occurs. Local anaesthetics are 'use dependent'; that is, the degree of block is proportional to the rate of nerve stimulation. This indicates that more drug molecules (in their protonated form) enter the Na^+ channels when they are open and cause more inactivation. This property is particularly important in the antiarrhythmic action of local anaesthetics (Chapter 17).

CHEMISTRY

Commonly used local anaesthetics consist of a lipophilic end (often an aromatic ring) and a hydrophilic end (usually a secondary or tertiary amine) connected by an intermediate chain that incorporates an ester or amide linkage.

EFFECTS

These may be: (1) *local* and include nerve blockade and direct effects on vascular smooth muscle; (2) *regional*, comprising loss of sensations (pain, temperature, touch) and vasomotor tone in the region supplied by the blocked nerves; and (3) *systemic* effects occurring because of absorption or intravenous administration.

Heart. The effects of local anaesthetics on the *heart* are discussed in Chapter 17. Cardiac toxicity probably does not occur in subconvulsive doses.

Vascular smooth muscle. The local effects vary. *Cocaine* is a vasoconstrictor (because it blocks noradrenaline reuptake and potentiates sympathetic activity) whilst *procaine* is a vasodilator. Most *amides* cause vasoconstriction at low concentrations and vasodilatation at higher concentrations. Prilocaine is most likely to produce vasoconstriction at clinical doses followed by lignocaine and bupivacaine. The regional effect is vasodilatation caused by blockade of sympathetic nerves.

Duration of action. In general, high potency and long duration are related to high lipid solubility because this results in much of the locally applied drug entering the cells. Vasoconstriction also tends to prolong the anaesthetic effect by reducing systemic distribution of the agent and this can be achieved by the addition of a vasoconstrictor such as adrenaline, noradrenaline or felypressin (a peptide). Vasoconstrictors must not be used for producing ring-block of an extremity (e.g. finger or toe) because they may cause prolonged ischaemia and gangrene.

Amides are dealkylated in the liver and esters (not cocaine) are hydrolysed by plasma pseudocholinesterase, but drug metabolism has little effect on the duration of action of agents actually in the tissues.

METHODS OF ADMINISTRATION

Surface anaesthesia. Topical application to external or mucous surface.

Infiltration anaesthesia. Subcutaneous injection to act on local nerve endings, usually with a vasoconstrictor.

Nerve block. Techniques range from infiltration of anaesthetic around a single nerve (e.g. dental anaesthesia) to epidural and spinal anaesthesia. In spinal anaesthesia (intrathecal block) a drug is injected into the cerebrospinal fluid in the subarachnoid space. In epidural anaesthesia, the anaesthetic is injected outside the dura. Spinal anaesthesia is technically far easier to produce than epidural anaesthesia, but the latter technique virtually eliminates the post-anaesthetic complications such as headache.

Intravenous regional anaesthesia. Anaesthetic is injected intravenously into an exsanguinated limb. A tourniquet prevents the agent reaching the systemic circulation.

6 Drugs acting at the neuromuscular junction

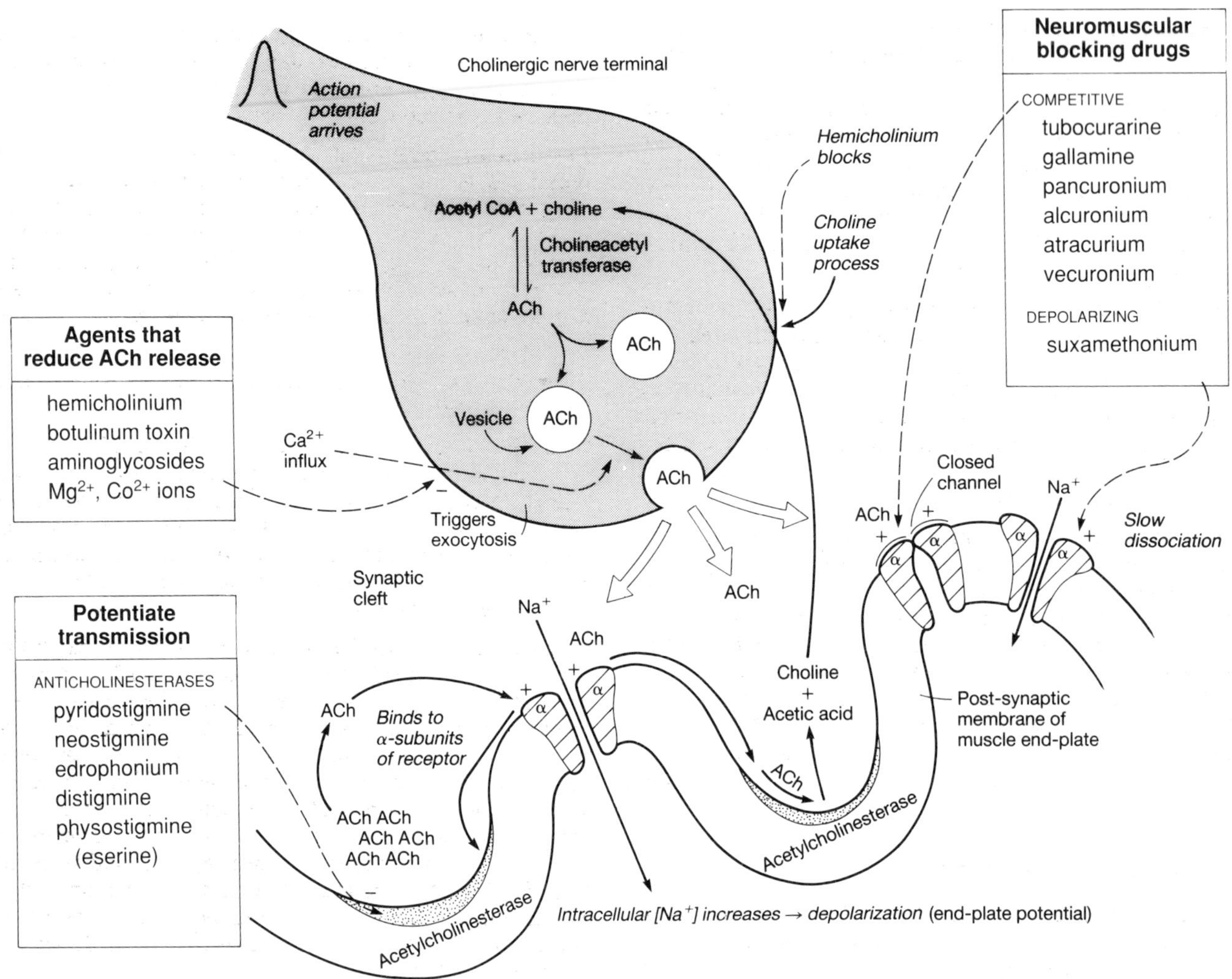

Action potentials are conducted along the motor nerves to their terminals (upper figure, ▒) where the depolarization initiates an influx of Ca^{2+} ions and the release of **acetylcholine** (ACh) by a process of **exocytosis** (⇨). The acetylcholine diffuses across the junctional cleft and binds to **receptors** located on the surface of the muscle-fibre membrane at the motor end-plate. The reversible combination of acetylcholine and receptors (lower figure, ▨) triggers the opening of cation-selective channels in the end-plate membrane, allowing an influx of Na^+ ions and a lesser efflux of K^+ ions. The resulting depolarization, which is called an end-plate potential (EPP), depolarizes the adjacent muscle-fibre membrane. If large enough, this depolarization results in an action potential and muscle contraction. The acetylcholine released into the synaptic cleft is rapidly hydrolysed by an enzyme, acetylcholinesterase (░), which is present in the end-plate membrane close to the receptors.

Neuromuscular transmission can be increased by **anticholinesterase drugs** (bottom left) which inhibit acetylcholinesterase and slow down the hydrolysis of acetylcholine in the synaptic cleft (see also Chapter 8). *Neostigmine* and *pyridostigmine* are used in the treatment of **myasthenia gravis** and to reverse competitive neuromuscular blockade after surgery. Overdosage of anticholinesterases results in excess acetylcholine and a depolarization block of motor end-plates (cholinergic weakness). The muscarinic effects of acetylcholine (see Chapter 7) are also potentiated by anticholinesterases but are blocked with atropine.

Neuromuscular blocking drugs (right) are used by anaesthetists to relax skeletal muscles during surgical operations and to prevent muscle contractions during electroconvulsive therapy (ECT). Most of the clinically useful neuromuscular blocking drugs compete with acetylcholine for the receptor but do not initiate ion channel opening. These '**competitive**' drugs reduce the end-plate depolarizations produced by acetylcholine to a size which is below the threshold for muscle action potential generation and so cause a flaccid paralysis. **Depolarizing blockers** also act on acetylcholine receptors, but trigger the opening of the ion channels. They are not reversed by anticholinesterases. *Suxamethonium* is the only drug of this type used clinically.

Some agents (top left) act **presynaptically** and block neuromuscular transmission by preventing the release of acetylcholine.

Acetylcholine is synthesized in motoneurone terminals from choline and acetylcoenzyme-A by the enzyme choline acetyltransferase. The choline is taken up into the nerve endings from the extracellular fluid by a special choline carrier located in the terminal membrane.

Exocytosis. Acetylcholine is stored in nerve terminals in the cytoplasm and within synaptic vesicles (each vesicle containing about 10 000 acetylcholine molecules). When an action potential invades the terminal, Ca^{2+} ions enter and cause the vesicles to collide with the outer terminal membrane. This results in the release of a few hundred 'packets' or 'quanta' of acetylcholine in about a millisecond. This is called quantal release and is very sensitive to the extracellular Ca^{2+} ion concentration. Divalent ions, such as Mg^{2+}, Co^{2+} and Mn^{2+}, antagonize Ca^{2+} influx and inhibit transmitter release.

Acetylcholine receptor. This can be activated by nicotine and for this reason is called a **nicotinic receptor**[1]. The receptor–channel complex is constructed from four different protein subunits (denoted β, γ, δ and 2 αs) which span the membrane and are arranged to form a central pore (channel) through which cations (mainly Na^+) flow. Acetylcholine molecules bind to the two α-subunits inducing a conformational change that opens the channel for about 1 millisecond.

Myasthenia gravis is an autoimmune disease in which neuromuscular transmission is defective. Circulating heterogeneous immunoglobulin G (IgG) antibodies cause a loss of functional acetylcholine receptors in skeletal muscle. To counteract the loss of or damage to receptors, the amount of acetylcholine in the synaptic cleft is increased by the administration of an anticholinesterase. Immunological treatment includes administration of prednisolone or azathioprine (Chaper 40). Plasmaphoresis, in which blood is removed and the cells returned, may improve motor function, presumably by reducing the level of immune complexes. Thymectomy may be curative.

PRESYNAPTIC AGENTS

Drugs affecting acetylcholine synthesis. Certain analogues of choline (e.g. *hemicholinium*) inhibit choline uptake into the nerve terminals, causing a depletion of acetylcholine and a failure of its transmission: such drugs have a very slow onset because of the time taken for the acetylcholine stores to run down and they have no clinical use.

Drugs inhibiting acetylcholine release. *Botulinum toxin* is produced by *Clostridium botulinum* (an anaerobic bacillus, see Chapter 35). The exotoxin is extraordinarily potent and prevents acetylcholine release by an unknown mechanism. *C. botulinum* is very rarely responsible for serious food poisoning in which the victims exhibit progressive parasympathetic and motor paralysis.

Recently, botulinium toxin type A has been found to be of value in the treatment of certain dystonias, such as blepharospasm (spasmodic eye closure) and strabismus (squint). In these conditions, low doses of toxin are injected into the appropriate muscle to produce paralysis which persists for about 12 weeks.

Aminoglycoside antibiotics (e.g. gentamicin) may cause neuromuscular blockade by inhibiting the calcium influx required for exocytosis. This unwanted effect usually only occurs as the result of an interaction with neuromuscular blockers. Myasthenia gravis may be exacerbated.

[1] Nicotinic receptors also occur in autonomic ganglia and the brain. They have a different subunit construction and pharmacology.

COMPETITIVE NEUROMUSCULAR BLOCKING DRUGS

These all have one or more protonated N atoms and do not pass the blood–brain barrier. They are administered by intravenous injection.

Tubocurarine acts for about 40 minutes and is excreted largely unchanged by the kidneys. It partly blocks ganglionic transmission causing hypotension. It may cause histamine release and occasionally hypersensitivity reactions.

Pancuronium is a steroidal neuromuscular blocking drug with a duration of action of about 40 minutes but with a swifter onset of action than tubocurarine. It does not block ganglia, causes minimal histamine release and has largely replaced tubocurarine as the drug of choice in major surgery. It has a dose-related, atropine-like effect on the heart and large doses may increase the work of the heart by increasing peripheral resistance.

Alcuronium has a duration of action of about 20 minutes, but is very dose dependent.

Gallamine does not block ganglia or release histamine but causes undesirable tachycardia by blocking the (M_2-muscarinic) heart acetylcholine receptors. These receptors are different from other muscarinic receptors and gallamine does not block muscarinic receptors in other organs (Chapter 7). Gallamine is excreted by the kidney and its use should be avoided in patients with severe renal disease.

Vecuronium and atracurium were found during a search for a successor to suxamethonium (see below). Such a drug was required to have a rapid onset without fasciculation, short predictable duration of action without the need for reversal agents and no autonomic effects. *Vecuronium* has fewest cardiovascular effects. It depends on hepatic inactivation and recovery can occur within 15–30 minutes making it an attractive drug for short procedures. *Atracurium* is an interesting compound which is only stable when kept cold and at low pH. At body pH and temperature it decomposes spontaneously in plasma and therefore does not depend on renal or hepatic function for its elimination. Atracurium has a duration of action of 15–30 minutes.

DEPOLARIZING NEUROMUSCULAR BLOCKING DRUGS

Suxamethonium (succinylcholine) is used because of its rapid onset and very short duration of action (3–7 minutes). The drug is normally hydrolysed rapidly by plasma pseudocholinesterase, but a few people inherit an atypical form of the enzyme and in such indivuals, the neuromuscular block may last for hours. Suxamethonium depolarizes the end-plate and because the drug does not dissociate rapidly from the receptors, a prolonged receptor activation is produced. The resulting end-plate depolarization initially causes a brief train of muscle action potentials and muscle-fibre twitches. Neuromuscular block then occurs as a result of several factors which include: (1) inactivation of the voltage-sensitive Na^+ channels in the surrounding muscle-fibre membrane, so that action potentials are no longer generated; and (2) transformation of the activated receptors to a 'desensitized' state, unresponsive to acetylcholine. The main disadvantage of suxamethonium is that the initial asynchronous muscle-fibre twitches cause damage which often results in muscle pains the next day. The damage also causes potassium release. Repeated doses of suxamethonium may cause bradycardia in the absence of atropine (a muscarinic effect).

7 Autonomic nervous system

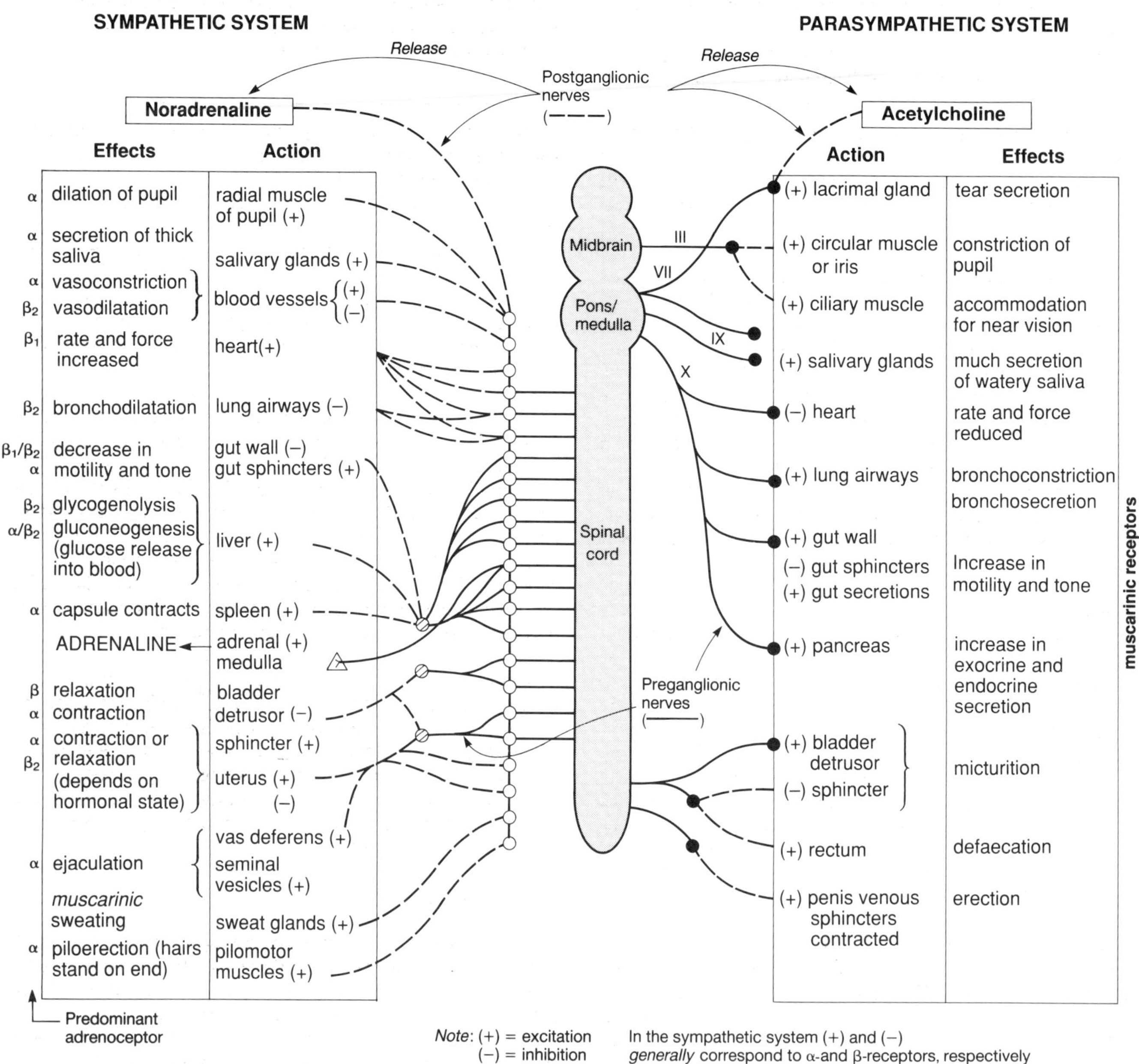

Note: (+) = excitation
(–) = inhibition

In the sympathetic system (+) and (–) *generally* correspond to α-and β-receptors, respectively

Many systems of the body (e.g. digestion, circulation) are controlled automatically by the autonomic nervous system (and the endocrine system). Control of the autonomic nervous system often involves negative feedback and there are many afferent (sensory) fibres which carry information to centres in the hypothalamus and medulla. These centres control the outflow of the autonomic nervous system, which is divided on anatomical grounds into two major divisions: the **sympathetic system** (left) and the **parasympathetic system** (right). Many organs are innervated by both systems, which in general have opposing actions. The actions of sympathetic (left) and parasympathetic (right) stimulation on different tissues are indicated in the inner columns and the resulting effects on different organs are shown in the outer columns.

The sympathetic nerves (left, ——) leave the thoracolumbar region of the spinal cord (T1-L3) and synapse either in the **paravertebral ganglia** (○), or in the **prevertebral ganglia** (⊘) and plexuses in the abdominal cavity. Postganglionic nonmyelinated nerve fibres (left, ----) arising from neurones in the ganglia, innervate most organs of the body (left).

The transmitter substance released at sympathetic nerve endings is **noradrenaline** (top left). Inactivation of this transmitter is largely by reuptake into the nerve terminals. Some preganglionic sympathetic fibres pass directly to the adrenal medulla (△) which can release adrenaline into the circulation. Noradrenaline and adrenaline produce their actions on effector organs by acting on **α-, β_1- or β_2-adrenoceptors** (extreme left).

In the parasympathetic system, the preganglionic fibres (right, ——) leave the central nervous system via the cranial nerves (especially III, VII, IX and X) and the third and fourth sacral spinal roots. They often travel much further than sympathetic fibres before synapsing in ganglia (●) which are often in the tissue itself (right).

The nerve endings of the postganglionic parasympathetic fibres (right, ----) release **acetylcholine** (top right), which produces its actions on the effector organs (right) by activating muscarinic receptors. Acetylcholine released at synapses is inactivated by the enzyme acetylcholinesterase.

All the preganglionic nerve fibres (sympathetic and parasympathetic, ——) are myelinated and release acetylcholine from the nerve terminals which depolarizes the ganglionic neurones by activating nicotinic receptors.

Adrenaline mimics most sympathetic effects, i.e. it is a *sympathomimetic agent* (Chapter 9). Elliot suggested in 1904 that adrenaline was the sympathetic transmitter substance, but Dale pointed out in 1910 that *noradrenaline* mimicked sympathetic nerve stimulation more closely.

Effects of sympathetic stimulation. These are most easily remembered by thinking of what changes in the body are appropriate in the '*fright or flight reaction*'. Note which effects are excitatory and which are inhibitory: (1) pupillary dilation (more light reaches the retina); (2) bronchiolar dilatation (facilitates increased ventilation); (3) heart rate and force are increased, blood pressure rises (more blood for increased activity of skeletal muscles—running!); (4) vasoconstriction in skin and viscera and vasodilatation in skeletal muscles (appropriate redistribution of blood to muscles), (5) contraction of spleen (provides more blood); and (6) to provide extra energy, glycogenolysis is stimulated and blood glucose level increases. The gastrointestinal tract and urinary bladder relax.

Adrenoceptors are divided into two main types: *α-receptors* mediate the excitatory effects of sympathomimetic amines, whilst their inhibitory effects are generally mediated by *β-receptors* (exceptions are the smooth muscle of the gut, where α-stimulation is inhibitory, and the heart, where β-stimulation is excitatory). Responses mediated by α-receptors and β-receptors can be distinguished: (1) by phentolamine and propranolol, which *selectively* block α- and β-receptors repectively; and (2) by the relative potencies, on different tissues, of noradrenaline (NA), adrenaline (A) and isoprenaline (I). The order of potency is NA > A > I where excitatory (α) responses are examined, but for inhibitory (β) responses this order is reversed (i.e. I ≫ A > NA).

β-Adrenoceptors are not homogeneous. For example, noradrenaline is an effective stimulant of cardiac β-receptors, but has little or no action on the β-receptors mediating vasodilatation. On the basis of the type of differential sensitivity they exhibit to drugs, β-receptors are divided into two types: β_1 (heart, intestinal smooth muscle) and β_2 (bronchial, vascular and uterine smooth muscle).

α-Adrenoceptors have been divided into two classes, originally depending on whether their location was post-synaptic (α_1) or presynaptic (α_2). Stimulation of the presynaptic α_2-receptors by synaptically released noradrenaline reduces further transmitter release (negative feedback). It is now clear that post-synaptic α_2-receptors occur in a few tissues, e.g. brain.

Acetylcholine is the transmitter substance released by:

1 All preganglionic autonomic nerves (i.e. both sympathetic and parasympathetic).
2 All postganglionic parasympathetic nerves.
3 Some postganglionic sympathetic nerves (i.e. thermoregulatory sweat glands and skeletal muscle vasodilator fibres).
4 Nerve to adrenal medulla.
5 Somatic motor nerves to skeletal muscle end-plates (Chapter 6).
6 Some neurones in the central nervous system (Chapter 21).

Acetylcholine receptors (cholinoreceptors) are divided into nicotinic and muscarinic subtypes (originally determined by measuring the sensitivity of various tissues to the drugs nicotine and muscarine respectively).

Muscarinic receptors. Acetylcholine released at the nerve terminals of postganglionic parasympathetic fibres acts on muscarinic receptors and can be blocked selectively by atropine. Three subtypes of muscarinic receptor exist, termed M_1, M_2 and M_3. M_1-receptors occur in the brain and gastric parietal cells, M_2-receptors in the heart and M_3-receptors in smooth muscle and glands. Except for **pirenzepine**, which selectively blocks M_1-receptors (Chapter 12), clinically useful muscarinic agonists and antagonists show little or no selectivity for the different subtypes of muscarinic receptor.

Nicotinic receptors occur in autonomic ganglia and in the adrenal medulla where the effects of acetylcholine (or nicotine) can be blocked selectively with hexamethonium. The nicotinic receptors at the skeletal muscle neuromuscular junction are not blocked by hexamethonium, but are blocked by tubocurarine. Thus receptors at ganglia and neuromuscular junctions are different, although both types are stimulated by nicotine and therefore called nicotinic.

Actions of acetylcholine

Muscarinic effects are mainly parasympathomimetic (except sweating and vasodilatation) and in general are the opposite to those caused by sympathetic stimulation. Muscarinic effects include: constriction of the pupil, accommodation for near vision (Chapter 10), profuse watery salivation, bronchiolar constriction, bronchosecretion, hypotension (due to bradycardia and vasodilatation), increase in gastrointestinal motility and secretion, contraction of the urinary bladder and sweating.

Nicotinic effects include stimulation of all autonomic ganglia. However, the action of acetylcholine on ganglia is relatively weak compared with its effect on muscarinic receptors and so parasympathetic effects predominate. The nicotinic actions of acetylcholine on the sympathetic system can be demonstrated, for example, on cat blood pressure, by blocking its muscarinic actions with atropine. High intravenous doses of acetylcholine then cause a rise in blood pressure, because stimulation of the sympathetic ganglia and adrenal medulla now result in vasoconstriction and tachycardia.

8 Autonomic drugs acting at cholinergic synapses

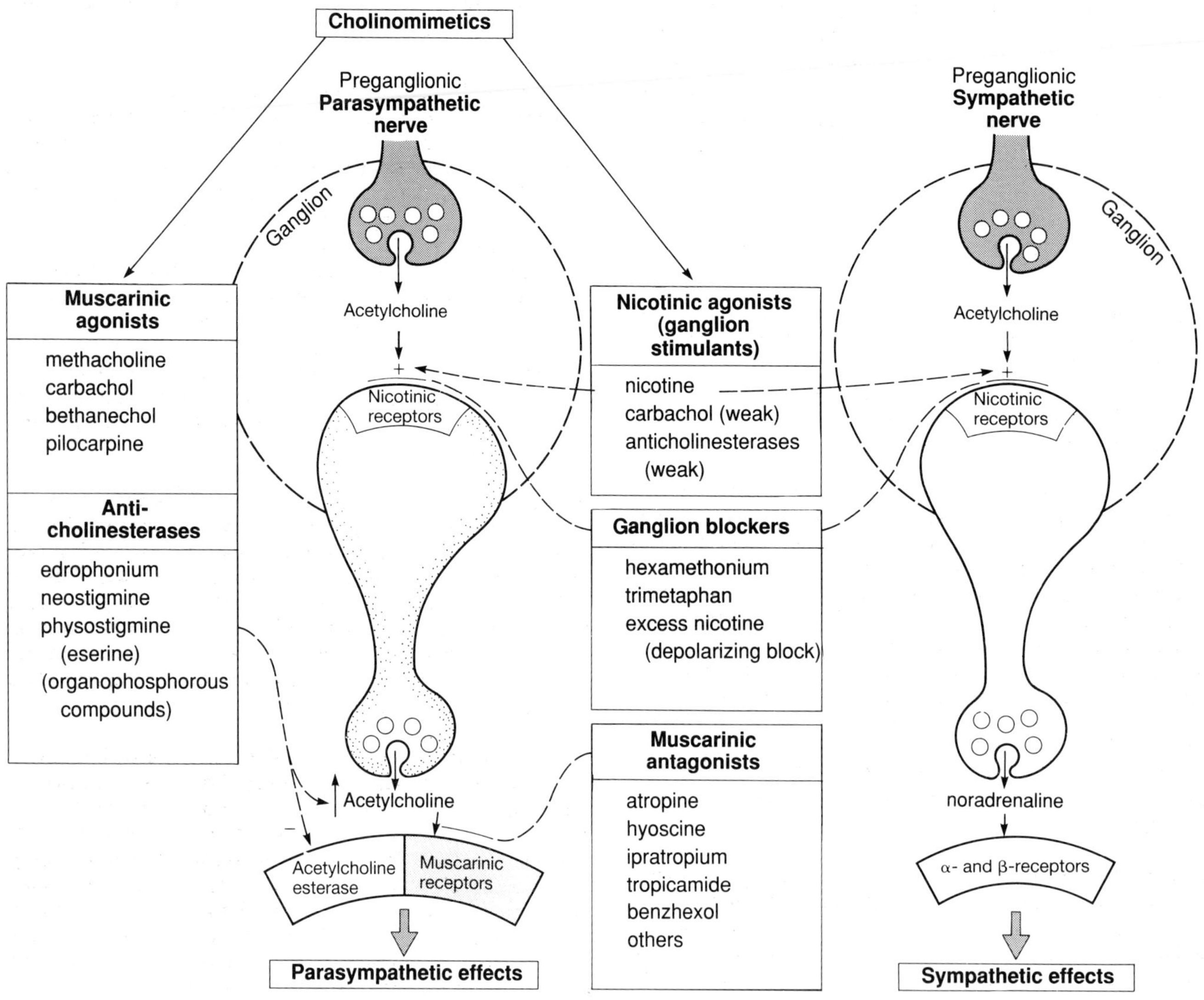

Acetylcholine released from the terminals of postganglionic parasympathetic nerves (left, ▒) produces its actions on various effector organs by activating **muscarinic receptors** (▭). The effects of acetylcholine are usually excitatory, but an important exception is the heart, which receives inhibitory cholinergic fibres from the vagus (Chapter 17). Drugs which mimic the effects of acetylcholine are called **cholinomimetics** and can be divided into two groups: (1) drugs that act directly on receptors (**nicotinic** and **muscarinic agonists**); and (2) **anticholinesterases**, which inhibit acetylcholinesterase, and so act indirectly by allowing acetylcholine to accumulate in the synapse and produce its effects.

Muscarinic agonists (top left) have relatively few uses, but *pilocarpine* (as eyedrops) is used to reduce intraocular pressure in glaucoma (Chapter 10). *Carbachol* or *bethanechol* are sometimes used to stimulate the gut in post-operative ileus and the bladder in urinary retention in conditions where there is no obstruction to the bladder outlet (e.g. in neurological disease or post-operatively).

Anticholinesterases (bottom left) have relatively little effect at ganglia and are used mainly for their nicotinic effects on the neuromuscular junction. They are used in the treatment of myasthenia gravis and to reverse the effects of competitive muscle relaxants used during surgery (Chapter 6).

Muscarinic antagonists (bottom middle) block the effects of acetylcholine released from postganglionic parasympathetic nerve terminals. Their effects can, in general, be worked out by examination of the figure in Chapter 7. However, parasympathetic effector organs vary in their sensitivity to the blocking effect of antagonists. Secretions of the salivary, bronchial and sweat glands are most sensitive to blockade. Higher doses of antagonist dilate the pupils, paralyse accommodation and produce tachycardia by blocking vagal tone in the heart. Still higher doses inhibit parasympathetic control of the gastrointestinal tract and bladder. Gastric acid secretion is most resistant to blockade (Chapter 12).

Atropine, *hyoscine* (scopolamine) or other antagonists are used: (1) in anaesthesia to block vagal slowing of the heart and to inhibit bronchial secretion; (2) to reduce intestinal spasm in, for example, irritable bowel syndrome; (3) to reduce gastric acid secretion (pirenzepine, Chapter 12); (4) in Parkinsonism (benzhexol, Chapter 25); (5) to prevent motion sickness (hyoscine); (6) to dilate the pupil for ophthalmological examination (e.g. tropicamide) or to paralyse the ciliary muscle (Chapter 10); and (7) as a bronchodilator in asthma (ipratropium, Chapter 11).

Transmission at autonomic ganglia (◌) can be stimulated by nicotinic agonists (top middle) or blocked by drugs that act specifically on the ganglionic neurone nicotinic receptor/ionophore (middle). They are of no clinical use because of their widespread effects.

Cholinergic nerve terminals in the autonomic nervous system synthesize, store and release acetylcholine in essentially the same way as at the neuromuscular junction (Chapter 6). Acctylcholinesterase is bound to both the pre- and post-synaptic membranes.

CHOLINOMIMETICS

Ganglion stimulants. These have widespread actions because they stimulate nicotinic receptors on both parasympathetic and sympathetic ganglionic neurones. Sympathetic effects include vasoconstriction, tachycardia and hypertension. Parasympathetic effects include increased motility of the gut and increased salivary and bronchial secretion. They have no clinical uses.

Muscarinic agonists. These directly activate muscarinic receptors, producing a variety of responses in different tissues. For example, in the heart, an increase in K^+ conductance causes bradycardia (Chapter 17), whilst a decrease in Ca^{2+} conductance reduces the force of contraction. Stimulation of smooth muscle receptors results in an increase in Na^+ conductance and contraction of the muscle. The mechanisms coupling muscarinic receptor activation with these different conductance changes are unclear. Activation of cardiac (M_2) receptors results in the inhibition of adenylyl cyclase which explains the negative inotropic effect of acetylcholine (Chapter 17). In other tissues, activation of muscarinic receptors (M_1, M_3) results in the formation of inositol triphosphate and increased cytosolic Ca^{2+} (Chapter 1).

Choline esters (methacholine, carbachol and bethanechol) are quaternary compounds, that do not penetrate the blood–brain barrier. Their actions are much more prolonged than acetylcholine, because they are either more resistant to hydrolysis by cholinesterase than acetylcholine (methacholine), or are not affected by the enzyme. Carbachol also stimulates nicotinic receptors.

Pilocarpine is an alkaloid that possesses a tertiary N atom which confers increased lipid solubility. This enables the drug to penetrate the cornea readily when applied locally and enter the brain when given systemically.

Effects of muscarinic agonists are generally the same as those produced by acetylcholine.

Anticholinesterases. These are indirectly acting cholinomimetics. The commonly used anticholinesterase drugs are quaternary compounds that do not pass the blood–brain barrier and have negligible central effects. They are poorly absorbed orally. Physostigmine (eserine) is a tertiary amine and is much more lipid soluble. It is well absorbed after oral or local administration (e.g. as eyedrops) and passes into the brain.

Mechanism of action. Initially, acetylcholine binds to the active site of the esterase and is hydrolysed producing free choline and acetylated enzyme. In a second step, the covalent acetyl–enzyme bond is split with the addition of water. *Edrophonium* is the main example of a reversible anticholinesterase. It binds by electrostatic forces to the active site of the enzyme. It does not form covalent bonds with the enzyme and so is very short acting (2–10 minutes). The carbamate esters (e.g. *neostigmine*, *pyridostigmine*) undergo the same two-step process as acetylcholine, except that the breakdown of the carbamylated enzyme is much slower (30 minutes–6 hours). Organophosphorous agents (e.g. *echothiophate*) result in a phosphorylated enzyme active site. The covalent phosphorus–enzyme bond is very stable and the enzyme is inactivated for hundreds of hours. For this reason, the organophosphorous compounds are referred to as irreversible anticholinesterases. They are extremely toxic and are used as insecticides (parathion malathion) and chemical warfare agents.

Effects of anticholinesterases are generally similar to those produced by the directly acting muscarinic agonists, but, in addition, transmission at the neuromuscular junction is potentiated. The cholinesterase inhibitors produce less vasodilatation than the directly acting agonists because they can only act on the (few) vessels possessing cholinergic innervation. Also, stimulation of sympathetic ganglia may oppose the vasodilator effects of the drug. Only large toxic doses of anticholinesterase produce marked bradycardia and hypotension.

Toxic doses initially cause signs of extreme muscarinic stimulation: miosis, salivation, sweating, bronchial constriction, bronchosecretion, vomiting and diarrhoea. Excessive stimulation of nicotinic receptors may cause depolarizing neuromuscular blockade. If the drug is lipid-soluble (e.g. physostigmine, organophosphorous compounds), convulsions, coma and respiratory arrest may occur. Strong nucleophiles (e.g. *pralidoxime*) can split the phosphorus–enzyme bond initially formed by organophosphorous compounds and 'regenerate' the enzyme. Later this becomes impossible because a process of 'ageing' strengthens the phosphorus–enzyme bond.

CHOLINERGIC RECEPTOR ANTAGONISTS

Ganglion blockers such as hexamethonium, are not simple competitive antagonists of acetylcholine, but also block the cation channel gated by the nicotinic receptor. Their effects include hypotension, mydriasis, dry mouth, anhidrosis, constipation, urinary retention and impotence.

Muscarinic antagonists. *Atropine* ((+), (−)-hyoscyamine) occurs in deadly nightshade (*Atropa belladonna*). It is a weak central stimulant, especially on the vagal nucleus and low doses often cause bradycardia. Higher doses cause tachycardia. (−)-Hyoscine (*scopolamine*) is more sedative than atropine and often produces drowsiness and amnesia. Toxic doses of both drugs cause excitement, agitation, hallucination and coma. The effects of muscarinic antagonists can be worked out by study of the figure in Chapter 7. The student should understand why these drugs produce dilated pupils, blurred vision, dry mouth, constipation and difficulty with micturition.

9 Drugs acting on the sympathetic system

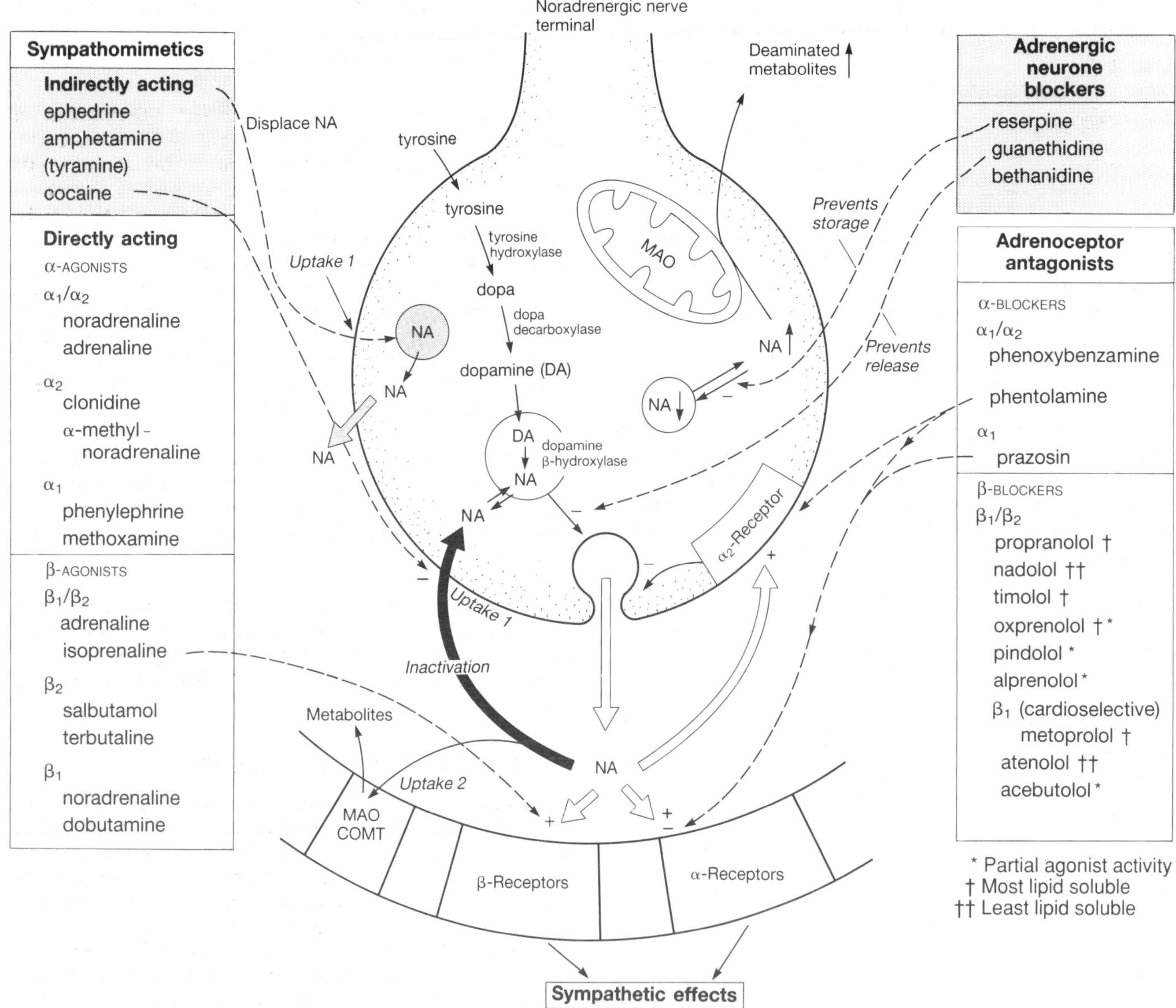

The sympathetic nervous system is important in regulating organs such as the heart and peripheral vasculature (Chapters 15 and 18). The transmitter released from sympathetic nerve endings is noradrenaline (⇨), but in response to some forms of stress adrenaline is also released from the adrenal medulla. These catecholamines are inactivated mainly by reuptake (➡).

Sympathomimetics (left) are drugs that partially or completely mimic the actions of noradrenaline and adrenaline. They act either **directly** on α- and/or β-adrenoceptors (left, open column) or **indirectly** on the presynaptic terminals (top left, shaded) usually by causing the release of noradrenaline (⇦). The effects of adrenoceptor stimulation can be seen in the figure in Chapter 7.

β₂-Adrenoceptor agonists cause bronchial dilatation and are used in the treatment of asthma (Chapter 11). They are also used to relax uterine muscle in an attempt to prevent preterm labour. **β₁-Adrenoceptor agonists** (dobutamine) are sometimes used to stimulate the force of heart contraction in severe low-output heart failure (Chapter 18). **α₁-Agonists** (e.g. phenylephrine) are used as mydriatics (Chapter 10) and in many popular decongestant preparations. **α₂-Agonists**, notably *clonidine* and *methyldopa* (which acts after its conversion to α-methylnoradrenaline, a false transmitter) are centrally acting hypotensive drugs (Chapter 15).

Sympathomimetic amines that act mainly by causing **noradrenaline release** (e.g. *amphetamine*) have the α/β selectivity of noradrenaline. *Ephedrine*, in addition to causing noradrenaline release, also has a direct action. Its effects resemble those of adrenaline, but they last much longer. Ephedrine is a mild central stimulant, but amphetamine, which enters the brain more readily, has a much greater stimulant effect on mood and alertness and a depressant effect on appetite. Amphetamine and similar drugs have a high abuse potential and are rarely used (Chapter 29).

β-Adrenoceptor antagonists (β-blockers) (bottom right) are important drugs used in the treatment of hypertension (Chapter 15), angina (Chapter 16), cardiac arrhythmias (Chapter 17), and glaucoma (Chapter 10). **α-Adrenoceptor antagonists (α-blockers)** (middle right) have limited clinical applications. *Prazosin*, a selective α_1-antagonist is sometimes used in the treatment of hypertension. *Phenoxybenzamine*, an irreversible antagonist, is used to block the α-effects of the large amounts of catecholamines released from tumours of the adrenal medulla (phaeochromocytoma). Many α-blockers have been (and are) used in the treatment of peripheral vascular occlusive disease, usually with little success.

Adrenergic neurone blocking drugs (top right, shaded) either deplete the nerve terminals of noradrenaline (reserpine) or prevent its release. They were used as hypotensive agents (Chapter 15).

Adrenergic nerve terminals contain vesicles where most of the noradrenaline is stored as a complex with ATP and protein (chromogranin). Vesicular noradrenaline is in equilibrium with cytoplasmic noradrenaline.

Uptake 1 is a high affinity transport process in the sympathetic nerve terminals. It 'recaptures' most of the released noradrenaline, and is the main method of terminating the actions of noradrenaline following its release into the synaptic cleft.

Uptake 2 is a similar transport process in the tissues but is less selective and less easily saturated.

MAO (monoamine oxidase) and **COMT (catechol-O-methyltransferase)** are widely distributed enzymes that catabolize catecholamines. Inhibition of MAO and COMT has little potentiating effect on responses to sympathetic nerve stimulation or injected catecholamines (noradrenaline, adrenaline) because they are largely inactivated by reuptake.

α_1-Adrenoceptors are post-synaptic. Their activation in several tissues (e.g. smooth muscle, salivary glands) causes an increase in inositol triphosphate and subsequently cytosolic calcium (Chapter 1) which triggers the response of the tissue.

α_2-Adrenoceptors occur on noradrenergic nerve terminals. Their activation by noradrenaline diminishes further transmitter release by a mechanism involving the inhibition of adenylyl cyclase and a reduced Ca^{2+} influx during the action potential.

β_1 and β_2-Adrenoceptor activation results in stimulation of adenylyl cyclase, increasing the conversion of ATP to cAMP. The cAMP acts as a 'second messenger' coupling receptor activation to response (Chapter 1).

SYMPATHOMIMETICS

Indirectly acting sympathomimetics displace noradrenaline from the storage vesicles of adrenergic nerves.

Amphetamine possesses an α-methyl group and is resistant to MAO. Its peripheral actions (e.g. tachycardia, hypertension) and central stimulant actions are mainly due to catecholamine release. D-amphetamine (dexamphetamine) is used in narcolepsy and sometimes in hyperkinetic children. Methylamphetamine, methylphenidate and phenmetrazine all have a high abuse potential, like amphetamine, and should not be used. Diethylpropion, dexfenfluramine, mazindol and phentermine have less central stimulant activity and are used as appetite suppressants in obesity. Dependence on these drugs is common (Chapter 29).

Cocaine, in addition to being a local anaesthetic (Chapter 5), is a sympathomimetic because it inhibits the reuptake of noradrenaline by nerve terminals. It has an intense central stimulant effect that has made it a popular drug of abuse (Chapter 29).

Directly acting sympathomimetics. The effect of sympathomimetic drugs in man depends on their receptor specificity (α and/or β) and on the compensatory reflexes they evoke.

Adrenaline and noradrenaline are destroyed in the gut and are short lasting when injected because of uptake and metabolism. Adrenaline increases the blood pressure by stimulating the rate and force of the heart beat (β_1-effects). Stimulation of vascular α-receptors causes vasoconstriction (viscera, skin) but β_2-stimulation causes vasodilatation (skeletal muscle) and the total peripheral resistance may actually decrease.

Noradrenaline has little or no effect on the vascular β_2-receptors and so the α-mediated vasoconstriction is unopposed. The resulting rise in blood pressure reflexively slows the heart, usually overcoming the direct β_1-stimulant action on heart rate.

Adrenaline by injection has an important use in the treatment of *anaphylactic shock* (Chapter 11).

β-Receptor selective drugs. *Isoprenaline* selectively stimulates β-receptors increasing the rate and force of the heart beat and causing vasodilatation. These effects result in a fall in diastolic and mean arterial pressure with little change in systolic pressure.

β_2-Adrenoceptor agonists are relatively selective drugs that produce bronchodilatation at doses that cause minimal effects on the heart. They are resistant to MAO and are probably not taken up into neurones. Their main use is in the treatment of asthma (Chapter 11).

ADRENOCEPTOR ANTAGONISTS

α-Blockers reduce arteriolar and venous tone, causing a fall in peripheral resistance and hypotension (Chapter 15). They reverse the pressor effects of adrenaline because its β_2-mediated vasodilator effects are unopposed by α-mediated vasoconstriction and the peripheral resistance falls (adrenaline reversal). α-Blockers cause a reflex tachycardia, which is greater with non-selective drugs that also block α_2-presynaptic receptors on the heart because the augmented release of noradrenaline stimulates further the cardiac β-receptors. *Prazosin*, a selective α_1-antagonist, causes relatively little tachycardia.

β-Blockers vary in their *lipid solubility* and *cardioselectivity*. However, they all block β_1-receptors and are equally effective in reducing blood pressure and preventing angina. The more lipid-soluble drugs are more rapidly absorbed from the gut, undergo more first-pass hepatic metabolism and are more rapidly eliminated. They are also more likely to enter the brain and cause central effects (e.g. bad dreams). *Cardioselectivity* is only relative and diminishes with higher doses. Nevertheless, selective β_1-blockade seems to produce less peripheral vasoconstriction (cold hands and feet) and does not reduce the response to exercise-induced hypoglycaemia (stimulation of gluconeogenesis in the liver is mediated by β_2-receptors). Cardioselective drugs may have sufficient β_2-activity to precipitate severe bronchospasm in patients with asthma and they should avoid β-blockers. Some β-blockers possess *intrinsic sympathomimetic activity* (i.e. are partial agonists, Chapter 2). The clinical importance of this is debatable, but see Chapter 16.

10 Ocular pharmacology

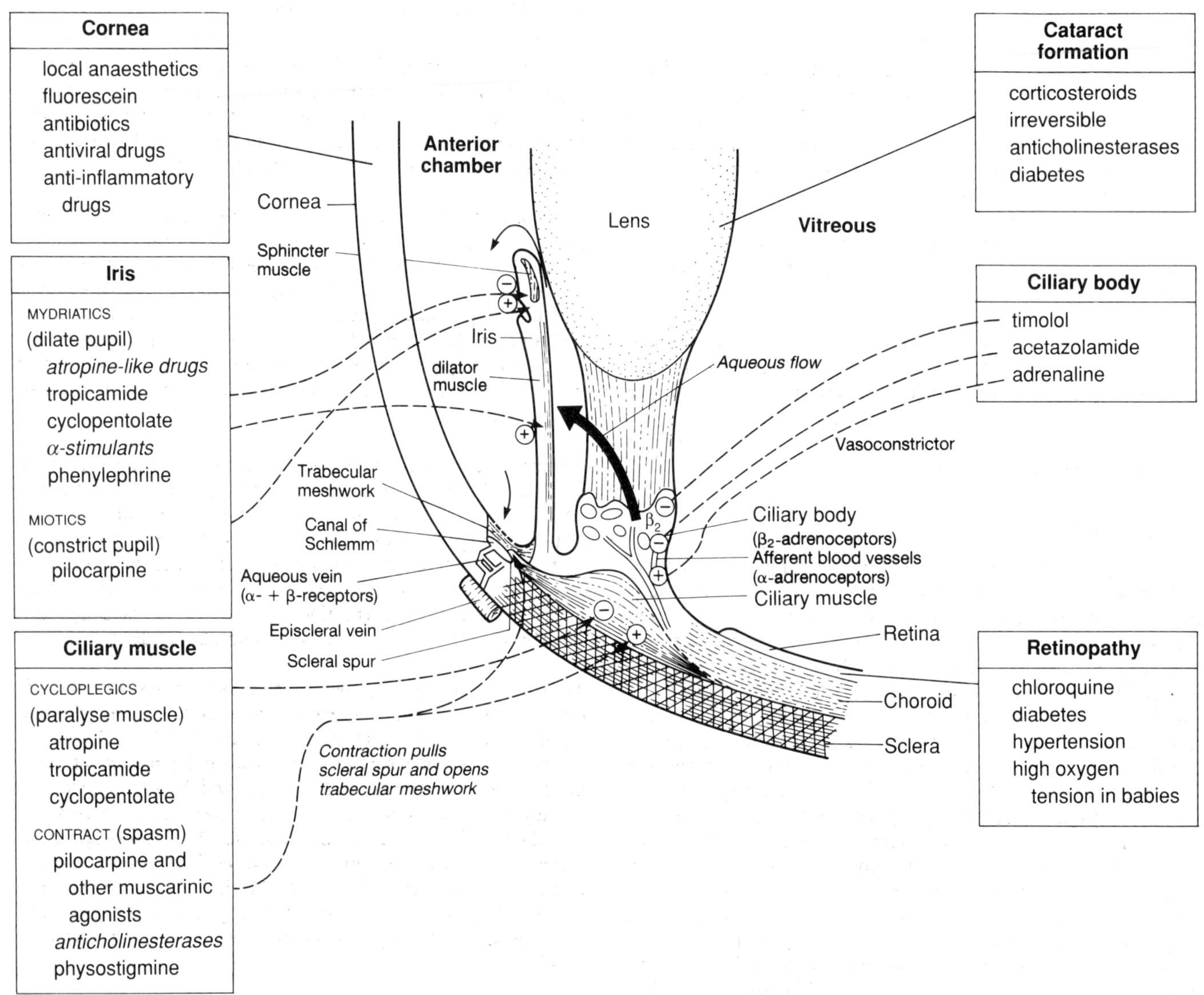

The eye is an inflated spherical shell, its outer layer being the tough, collagen-rich, sclera. The normal **intraocular pressure** (IOP) is about 15 mmHg and is maintained by a balance of aqueous humour formation by the *ciliary body* (⬅), and outflow through the *trabecular meshwork* into the canal of Schlemm (→). In open-angle **glaucoma** the IOP remains above 24 mmHg because pathological changes in the trabecular meshwork decrease the outflow of aqueous. Since the elevated IOP will eventually damage the optic nerve, the pressure must be reduced, usually with drugs. This can be done either by increasing aqueous outflow with **muscarinic agonists** such as *pilocarpine* (bottom left) or by reducing aqueous formation with a variety of drugs (middle right) but especially *timolol*, a β-blocker.

At the front of the eye, the sclera runs into the **cornea** (top left) whose transparency is obtained by alignment of the collagen fibres. Many superficial manipulations such as tonometry (measurement of the intraocular pressure) and the removal of corneal foreign bodies require the instillation of a *local anaesthetic*. *Fluorescein* is commonly instilled into the eye to reveal damaged areas of corneal epithelium, which are stained bright green by the dye. **Inflammation** of the cornea resulting from allergy or chemical burns is treated with topical anti-inflammatory drugs (Chapter 31). Infections are not treated with anti-inflammatory agents except together with an effective chemotherapeutic agent. This is because anti-inflammatory drugs reduce resistance to invading micro-organisms.

The **iris** (middle left) possesses a sphincter muscle, which receives parasympathetic nerves, and a dilator muscle, which is innervated by sympathetic fibres. Thus, muscarinic antagonists and α-adrenoceptor agonists *dilate* the pupil (**mydriasis**), whilst muscarinic agonists and α-adrenoceptor antagonists *constrict* the pupil (**miosis**).

Contraction of the parasympathetically innervated **ciliary muscle** (bottom left) allows the lens to become thicker and accommodation for near vision occurs. Thus, muscarinic antagonists *paralyse* the ciliary muscle (**cycloplegia**) and prevent accommodation for near vision, whilst agonists cause accommodation and a loss of far vision.

The **lens** (middle top) provides the adjustable part of the eye's refractive power. Opacity of the lens is called a cataract. Some drugs, notably corticosteroids, may cause cataracts.

The retina is a part of the central nervous system but it seems little affected by drugs, probably because of the effective blood–retinal barrier. The retina may be occasionally damaged by drugs, (e.g. chloroquine, quinine, ethambutol) or by high oxygen tension in newborn babies.

Ciliary body. The processes of the ciliary body are highly vascularized and are the sites of aqueous humour formation. The ciliary epithelial cells, which contain ATPase and carbonic anhydrase, absorb Na^+ selectively from the stroma and transport it into the intercellular clefts, which open only on the aqueous humour side. The hyperosmolality in the clefts causes water flow from the stroma producing a continuous flow of aqueous. The ciliary epithelium is leaky, allowing significant passive filtration, and up to 30% of aqueous may be formed by ultrafiltration.

Trabecular meshwork. The aqueous humour circulates through the pupil and is drained into the canal of Schlemm, which is a circular gutter within the surface of the sclera at the limbus. The sieve-like trabecular meshwork is the roof of the gutter, through which the aqueous must pass before it is eventually drained away into the episcleral veins.

GLAUCOMA

This is a group of ocular diseases with the common features of abnormally high IOP and ultimate loss of vision if untreated. It occurs in about 1% of people over 40 years of age. Viewed through an ophthalmoscope, the optic disc appears depressed (cupping) because of the loss of nerve fibres. The mechanism by which the nerve fibres are destroyed in glaucoma is unclear, but may involve mechanical factors and/or local ischaemia. Open-angle (chronic simple) glaucoma is the most common form of the disease. In closed-angle glaucoma, the angle between the cornea and the iris is abnormally small. Occasionally, the angle closes completely, preventing aqueous outflow, and the IOP quickly rises. Since permanent damage to the retina can occur during these attacks, the pressure must be reduced as quickly as possible by intensive instillation of pilocarpine eyedrops combined if necessary with intravenous *acetazolamide* and intravenous hypertonic mannitol (an osmotic agent), to remove water. Acetazolamide inhibits carbonic anhydrase in the ciliary body and prevents bicarbonate synthesis. This leads to a fall in sodium transport and aqueous formation because bicarbonate and sodium transport are linked.

Pilocarpine, being a tertiary amine, diffuses readily through the cornea into the aqueous humour. It reduces the IOP by contracting the ciliary muscle. This pulls the scleral spur and results in the trabecular meshwork being stretched and separated. The fluid pathways are opened up and aqueous outflow is increased.

Physostigmine is rarely used in glaucoma because of contact sensitivity reactions. Irreversible anticholinesterases, such as echothiophate, are associated with a high degree of cataract formation.

All parasympathomimetics cause miosis, resulting in poor night vision and complaints of 'dimming of vision'. Accommodation spasm that increases near-sightedness causing blurred vision is not usually a problem in the age group that develops glaucoma. Some patients find these effects intolerable.

Timolol is the drug of choice in open-angle glaucoma. It blocks β_2-adrenoceptors on the ciliary processes and so reduces aqueous secretion. In addition, timolol may block β-receptors in the afferent blood vessels supplying the ciliary processes. The resulting vasoconstriction results in reduced ultrafiltration and aqueous formation. Timolol avoids the unpleasant effects of pilocarpine on the eye, but it is absorbed systemically and may provoke bronchospasm in asthmatics or bradycardia in susceptible patients.

Adrenaline and α-adrenoceptor stimulants lower the IOP by an α-mediated vasoconstriction of the ciliary body afferent blood vessels. Confusingly, α-antagonists and β-adrenoceptor agonists (especially β_2-stimulants) also lower the IOP. These drugs increase the outflow of aqueous rather than reducing its formation, presumably by dilatation of the aqueous veins and/or episcleral veins. **Guanethidine** increases and prolongs the actions of adrenaline by blocking its uptake by the tissues.

Alternative to drugs in glaucoma. A recently introduced technique is laser trabecular surgery. Under local anaesthesia, the surgeon uses an argon laser to place about 100 evenly spaced lesions on the inner surface of the trabecular meshwork. The laser 'burns' cause localized shrinkage, which exerts tension on the adjacent, untreated tissue, opening spaces in the meshwork and allowing increased aqueous drainage. In closed-angle glaucoma, a YAG (yttrium aluminium garnet) laser may be used to make a hole at the periphery of the iris. This prevents the forward movement of the iris that precipitates acute glaucoma and is usually due to a partial block of aqueous flow through the pupil.

MYDRIATICS

Mydriasis (dilation of the pupil) is required for ophthalmoscopy. The drops most commonly used are the relatively short-acting muscarinic antagonists *tropicamide* and *cyclopentolate* which produce both mydriasis and cycloplegia. The α-adrenoceptor stimulant *phenylephrine* may be used to produce mydriasis without affecting the pupillary light reflex or accommodation. When the examination is complete, *physostigmine* or *pilocarpine* eyedrops can be given to antagonize the mydriatic, but this is only done very rarely. Phenylephrine mydriasis can be reversed with the α-antagonist, *thymoxamine*. Mydriasis may precipitate acute closed-angle glaucoma in susceptible patients who are usually aged over 60 years.

11 Asthma, hay fever and anaphylaxis

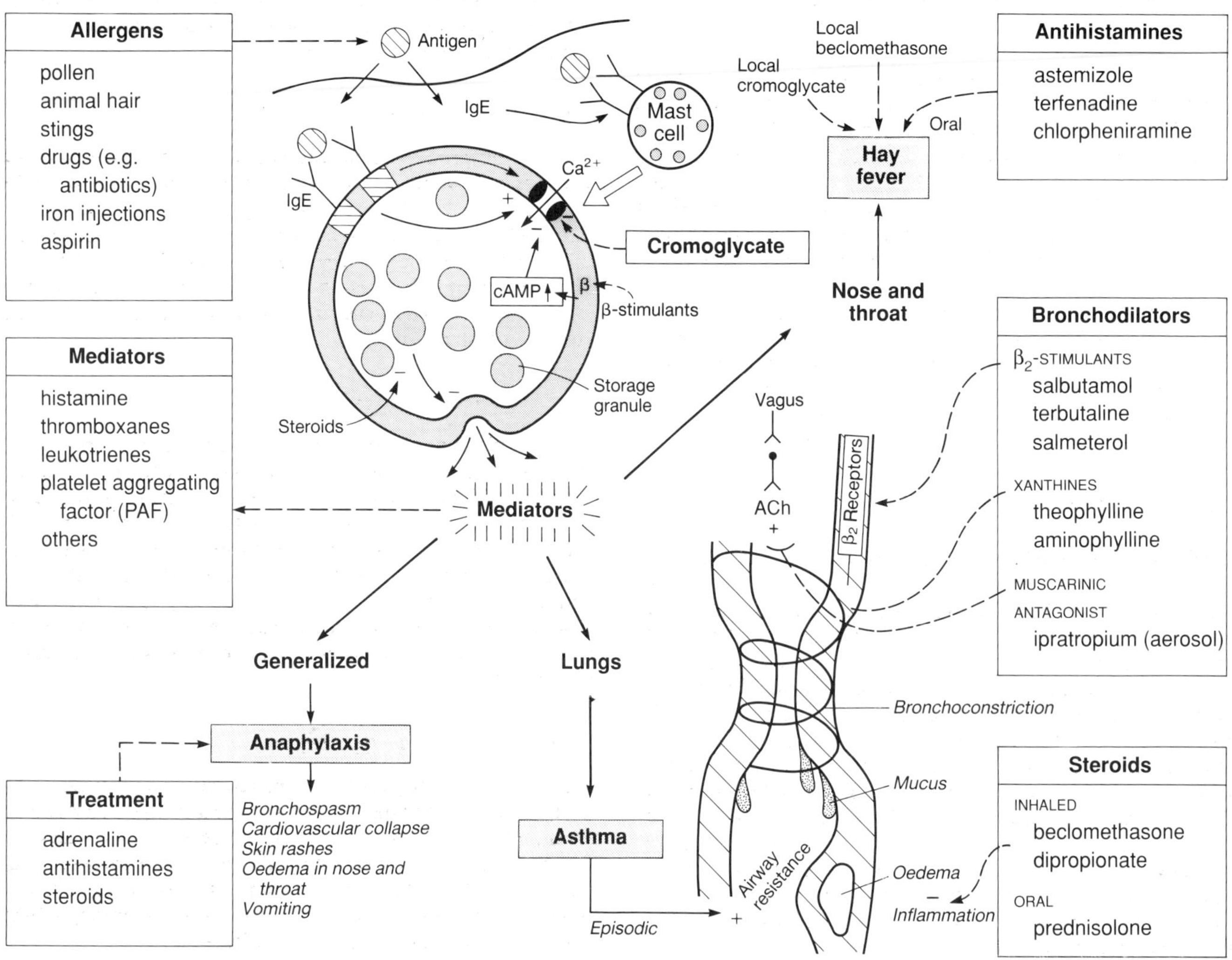

Asthma, hay fever and anaphylaxis (shaded boxes) are caused by the same basic processes: *IgE* antibody attaches to mast cells (top left), and on renewed exposure to the same antigen (⦸) degranulation of the mast cells occurs with the production and release of *mediators* (middle left). If the release of mediators is localized, hay fever (top right) or asthma (bottom right) result, but a massive general release causes anaphylaxis, which is a rare, but life-threatening, reaction to bee stings and penicillin or other drugs. Antigens that can trigger these reactions are called *allergens* (top left).

Bronchial asthma is an inflammatory disease in which the calibre of the airways is chronically narrowed by oedema and is unstable. During an attack the patient suffers from wheezing and difficulty in breathing due to bronchospasm, mucosal oedema and mucus formation (bottom right). When the acute attack has an allergic basis the term *extrinsic asthma* is often used. When there is no obvious allergic basis for the disease it is called *intrinsic asthma*.

In **mild to moderate asthma**, the first-line drugs are the *β_2-adrenoceptor agonists* (middle right), inhaled from pressurized containers. These drugs produce bronchodilatation via the production of cAMP which is presumed to somehow affect calcium in the bronchial smooth muscle causing relaxation. Inhaled *ipratropium* (a muscarinic antagonist), *steroids* and *cromoglycate* are important second-line drugs for patients whose asthma is not controlled using β_2-agonists alone. Oral preparations may be useful in patients with nocturnal wheezing and in children who cannot use inhalers. Oral *theophylline* is effective, but its toxicity and narrow therapeutic index are disadvantages. Some patients are only controlled by oral steroids (e.g. prednisolone, Chapter 31).

Acute severe attacks of asthma (status asthmaticus) which are not controlled by the patient's usual drugs are potentially fatal and must be dealt with as an emergency, requiring hospital admission.

IgE is the major class of reaginic antibody. In allergic patients, specific antibody levels may be increased to 100 times greater than normal. Binding of the F_c portion of the antibody to receptors on mast cells followed by cross-linking of adjacent molecules by antigen triggers degranulation by a mechanism involving Ca^{2+} influx.

Mast cells contain the body stores of histamine and occur in almost all tissues. Within the mast cells, histamine is bound with heparin and ATP in cytoplasmic granules. Histamine release normally involves an influx of Ca^{2+} ions and, because the permeability of the cell membrane to Ca^{2+} ions is reduced when intracellular cAMP levels are raised, drugs that either stimulate cAMP synthesis (β_2-adrenoceptor agonists) or prevent its breakdown (xanthines) reduce histamine release.

Mediators. It is not known which of the many possible mediators are released during an asthmatic attack and, since many of the mediators duplicate one another's actions, it is unlikely that a specific antagonist of one will be of therapeutic value. Hence the failure of antihistamines or aspirin (which blocks prostaglandin synthesis) to be useful in treating asthma.

BRONCHODILATORS

β-Adrenoceptor stimulants. The airway smooth muscle has few adrenergic nerve fibres but many β_2-receptors, stimulation of which causes bronchodilatation. β_2-Agonists such as **salbutamol** are usually given by inhalation. They are not specific, but β_1 effects (cardiac stimulation) are not usually seen at doses which cause bronchodilatation. Adverse effects include fine tremor, nervous tension and tachycardia, but these are not usually troublesome when the drug is given by inhalation. Oral administration is usually restricted to children and other patients who cannot use an aerosol preparation. **Salmeterol** is a new drug that is much longer lasting than salbutamol, but has a slower onset and is not intended for symptomatic relief. There is some evidence that inhaled β_2-agonists given regularly, rather than 'as necessary', cause asthma to deteriorate. The reason for this is not clear, but it has been suggested that prolonged bronchodilatation allows greater exposure to allergens or other factors which worsen asthma. Currently, more emphasis is being put on the earlier use of inhaled steroids.

Ipratropium is a muscarinic antagonist and an effective bronchodilator, presumably because it reduces reflex vagal bronchoconstriction which results from histamine stimulation of sensory (irritant) receptors in the airways. Ipratropium given by inhalation rarely causes atropine-like side-effects, such as dry mouth, and does not increase mucus viscosity or affect mucociliary clearance of sputum.

Xanthines often cause adverse effects, but there is growing use of oral sustained-release theophylline preparations which are effective for up to 12 hours. Even when plasma concentrations are in the therapeutic range (10–20 mg litre^{-1}), nausea, headache, insomnia and abdominal discomfort are common. Above 25 mg litre^{-1}, toxic effects include serious arrhythmias and convulsions which may be fatal. Theophylline may benefit children, who cannot use inhalants, and adults with predominantly nocturnal symptoms. It is not known how theophylline causes bronchodilatation in asthmatics. Xanthines inhibit phosphodiesterase and increase cellular cAMP levels but not at clinically effective concentrations. Theophylline is an antagonist at adenosine receptors, and as inhaled adenosine causes bronchoconstriction in asthmatics, this action may be important. However, it is not clear that adenosine has a pathophysiological role in asthma.

CROMOGLYCATE

This is a prophylactic drug and is of no value in acute attacks. It appears to be most effective in 'atopic' patients, especially children, sensitive to a wide variety of allergenic substances. Cromoglycate must be given regularly and it may be several weeks before beneficial effects are apparent. The mechanism of action of cromoglycate is unclear, but it reduces the influx of calcium into antigen-sensitized mast cells, and prevents the release of histamine.

GLUCOCORTICOIDS

Steroids effectively increase the airway calibre in asthma, but it is not known how. The drugs may act by reducing bronchial mucosal inflammatory reactions (e.g. oedema and mucus hypersecretion) and by modifying allergic reactions. Oral administration of steroids is associated with many serious adverse effects (Chapter 31), but these can be avoided in asthma by aerosol administration of the drugs (e.g. *beclomethasone dipropionate*). Inhaled steroids are usually effective in 3–7 days, but oral steroids may be necessary in some patients, where all other therapy fails.

ACUTE SEVERE ASTHMA

Oxygen is given together with nebulized or intravenous β_2-agonists (e.g. salbutamol). Then intravenous *hydrocortisone* is given, but this will not be effective for several hours (Chapter 31). Nebulized ipratropium may also be used if required, but may cause difficulty in micturition. If these drugs do not produce a response, an intravenous infusion of aminophylline may help. Artificial ventilation may be required.

ANTIHISTAMINES

Antagonists that block H_1-histamine receptors are used in the treatment of allergic conditions such as hay fever, urticaria, drug sensitivity rashes, pruritis and insect bites and stings. Older antihistamine drugs (e.g. chlorpheniramine, trimeprazine, promethazine) have antimuscarinic actions and pass the blood–brain barrier, commonly causing drowsiness and psychomotor impairment. Newer agents (e.g. astemizole, terfenadine) do not have atropine-like actions and because they do not cross the blood–brain barrier, they do not cause psychomotor impairment.

ANAPHYLAXIS

This requires prompt treatment with adrenaline, usually given by intramuscular injection (Chapter 9), followed by an antihistamine (e.g. chlorpheniramine) and corticosteriod (hydrocortisone) intravenously.

12 Drugs acting on the gastrointestinal tract: I peptic ulcer

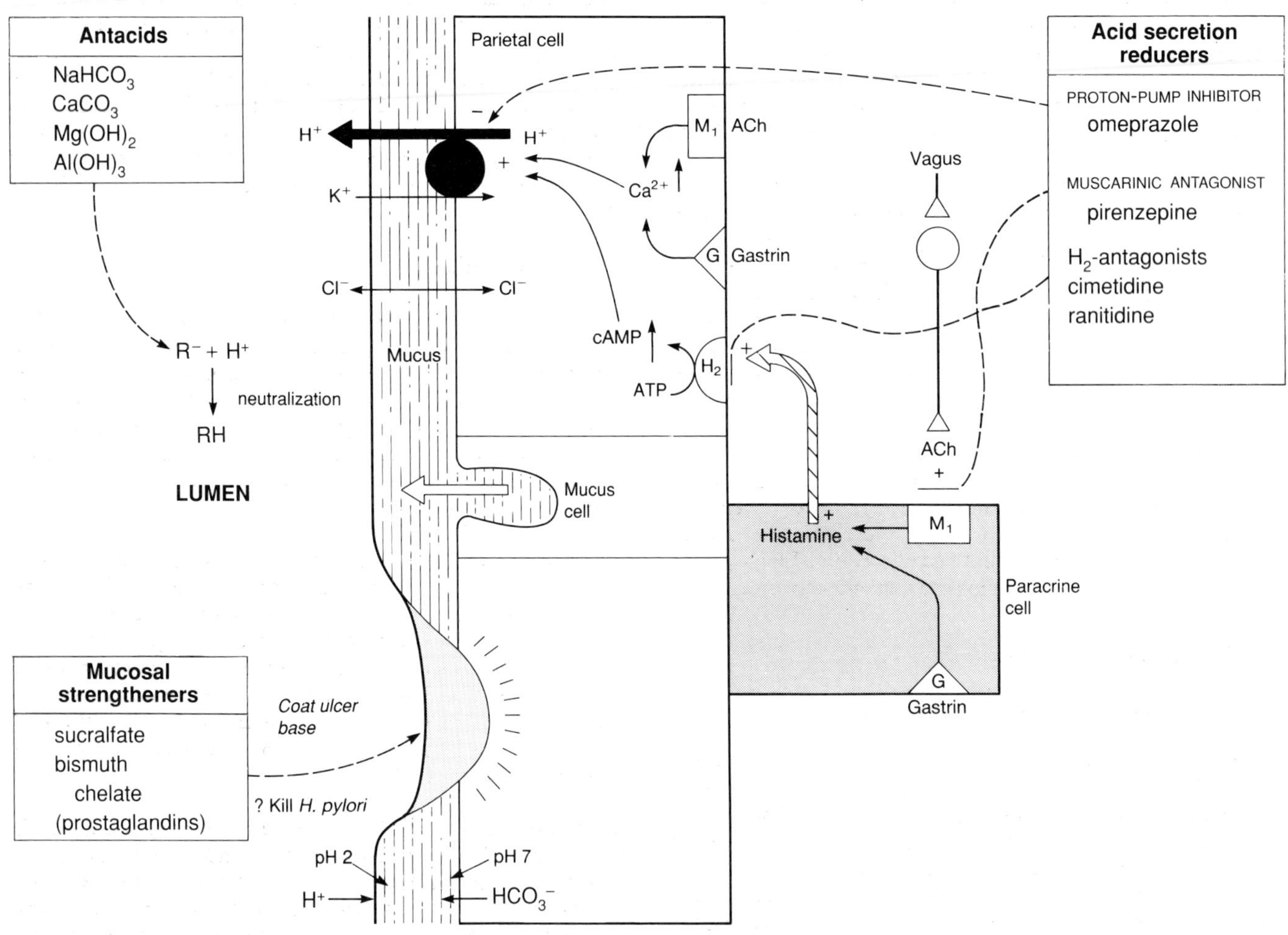

The term **peptic ulcer** refers to any ulcer in an area where the mucosa is bathed in the hydrochloric acid and pepsin of gastric juice (i.e. the stomach and upper part of the duodenum). Drugs that are effective in the treatment of peptic ulcer either **reduce gastric acid secretion** (right) or **increase mucosal resistance** to acid–pepsin attack (bottom left).

Acid secretion from the *parietal cells* (⬅) is reduced by **H_2-histamine antagonists** (*cimetidine, ranitidine*), which are the first-line drugs in ulcer treatment. *Pirenzepine*, a cholinergic M_1-muscarinic antagonist with a relatively selective action in the gut, also decreases acid secretion, but less effectively than the H_2-blockers, probably because it does not block gastrin-stimulated acid release. Nevertheless, the rate of healing with pirenzepine is comparable with that obtained with H_2-antagonists. *Omeprazole* can produce virtual antacidity by irreversibly inhibiting the proton pump (●), which transports H^+ ions out of the parietal cells. It is very effective in promoting ulcer healing, even in patients resistant to H_2-antagonists. The **'mucosal strengtheners'** *sucralfate* and *bismuth chelate* increase ulcer healing by binding to the ulcer base (left, □). This provides **physical protection** and allows the secretion of HCO_3^- to re-establish the pH gradient normally present in the mucus layer (▥) which originates from mucus-secreting cells (⇦).

Peptic ulcers, however healed, will often recur without continuous drug administration. There is evidence that the recurrence of ulcers is slower following bismuth chelate administration, but the reason for this is unknown. It may well be due to the antibacterial action of bismuth, because chronic infection of the stomach with *Helicobacter pylori* is probably an aetiological factor in ulcer formation.

Antacids (top left) are bases that raise the gastric luminal pH by neutralizing gastric acid (middle left). They provide effective treatment for many dyspepsias and symptomatic relief in peptic ulcer and oesophageal reflux. Many proprietary mixtures are available which usually contain magnesium or aluminium salts.

ACID SECRETION

Parietal cells secrete acid into the stomach lumen. This is achieved by a unique H^+/K^+ ATPase (proton pump) which catalyzes the exchange of intracellular H^+ for extracellular K^+. The secretion of HCl is stimulated by *acetylcholine* (ACh) released from vagal postganglionic fibres (right of figure) and *gastrin*, released into the bloodstream from G-cells in the antral mucosa when they detect amino acids and peptides (from food) in the stomach, and by gastric distension via local and long reflexes.

Although the parietal cells possess muscarinic (M_1) and gastrin receptors (G), both acetylcholine and gastrin mainly stimulate acid secretion indirectly, by releasing *histamine* from paracrine cells (right, □) located close to the parietal cells. Histamine then acts locally (⇦) on the parietal cells, where activation of histamine H_2-receptors (H_2) results in an increase in intracellular cAMP and the secretion of acid. Because acetylcholine and gastrin act indirectly by releasing histamine, the effects on acid secretion of both vagal stimulation and gastrin are reduced by H_2-receptor antagonists.

Cholinergic agonists can powerfully stimulate acid secretion in the presence of H_2-antagonists, indicating that ACh released from the vagus must have limited access to the parietal cell muscarinic receptors. Gastrin acting directly on the parietal cells has a weak effect on acid secretion, but this is greatly potentiated when the histamine receptors are activated.

ULCER HEALING DRUGS

Acid-secretion reducers

Histamine H_2-receptor antagonists. **Cimetidine and ranitidine** are rapidly absorbed orally. They block the action of histamine on the parietal cells and reduce acid secretion. These drugs relieve the pain of peptic ulcer and increase the rate of ulcer healing. The incidence of side-effects is low. Cimetidine has slight anti-androgenic actions, and rarely causes gynaecomastia. Cimetidine also binds to cytochrome P-450 and may reduce the hepatic metabolism of drugs (e.g. warfarin, phenytoin and theophylline).

Muscarinic antagonists. Pirenzepine reduces gastric acid secretion by selectively blocking M_1 muscarinic-receptors (presumably those on the histamine containing cells) and, because most of the peripheral effects of ACh involve M_2- and M_3-receptors, it decreases acid secretion at doses that rarely cause dry mouth, blurred vision or urinary problems. Non-selective muscarinic antagonists (e.g. atropine, propantheline) are ineffective at tolerable doses.

Omeprazole is inactive at neutral pH, but in acid it rearranges into two types of reactive molecule which react with sulphydryl groups in the H^+/K^+ ATPase (proton pump) responsible for transporting H^+ ions out of the parietal cells. Since the enzyme is irreversibly inhibited, acid secretion only resumes after the synthesis of new enzyme. It is particularly useful in patients with severe gastric acid hypersecretion due to Zollinger–Ellison syndrome, a rare condition caused by an islet-cell gastrin-secreting tumour of the pancreas, and in patients with reflux oesophagitis where severe ulceration is usually resistant to other drugs.

PROTECTIVE FACTORS

Mucus layer. This forms a physical barrier (approximately 500 μm thick) on the surface of the stomach and proximal duodenum, and consists of a mucus gel into which HCO_3^- is secreted. Within the gel matrix the HCO_3^- neutralizes acid diffusing from the lumen. This creates a pH gradient and the gastric mucosa is maintained at a neutral pH, even when the stomach contents are at pH 2. Prostaglandins E_2 and I_2 are synthesized by the gastric mucosa, where they are thought to exert a cytoprotective action by stimulating the secretion of mucus and bicarbonate, and by increasing the mucosal blood flow.

Mucosal strengtheners

Sucralfate is a complex substance formed from sulphated sucrose and aluminium hydroxide. The molecules polymerize below pH 4 to give a very sticky gel which adheres strongly to the base of ulcer craters. The gel presumably protects the ulcerated area by allowing the development of the normal pH gradient caused by the secretion of HCO_3^-. Sucralfate is about as effective as cimetidine in promoting ulcer healing and has very few side-effects.

Bismuth chelate may act in a similar way to sucralfate. It has a strong affinity for mucosal glycoproteins, especially in the necrotic tissue of the ulcer craters, which become coated in a protective layer of polymer–glycoprotein complex. However, bismuth salts eradicate the organism *Helicobacter pylori* and it may be this action which is responsible for ulcer healing. Bismuth may blacken the teeth and stools. Bismuth and sucralfate must be given on an empty stomach or they will complex with food proteins.

Misoprostol is a synthetic analogue of prostaglandin E_1. It promotes healing of peptic ulcers but side-effects, especially diarrhoea, make it unsuitable for this purpose. It seems that the beneficial effects of prostaglandin analogues are due to the decrease in acid secretion that they cause, rather than by any cytoprotective action they may have.

ANTACIDS

Antacids raise the luminal pH of the stomach. This increases the rate of emptying and so the effect of antacids is short. Gastrin release is increased and because this stimulates acid release, larger amounts of antacids are needed than would be predicted (acid rebound). Frequent high doses of antacids promote ulcer healing, but such treatment is rarely practical.

Sodium bicarbonate is the only useful water-soluble antacid. It acts rapidly but has a transient action and absorbed bicarbonate in high doses may cause systemic alkalosis.

Magnesium hydroxide and magnesium trisilicate are insoluble in water and have a fairly rapid action. Magnesium has a laxative effect and may cause diarrhoea.

Aluminium hydroxide has a relatively slower action. Al^{3+} ions form complexes with certain drugs (e.g. tetracyclines) and tend to cause constipation. Mixtures of magnesium and aluminium compounds may be used to minimize the effects on motility.

13 Drugs acting on the gastrointestinal tract: II motility and secretions

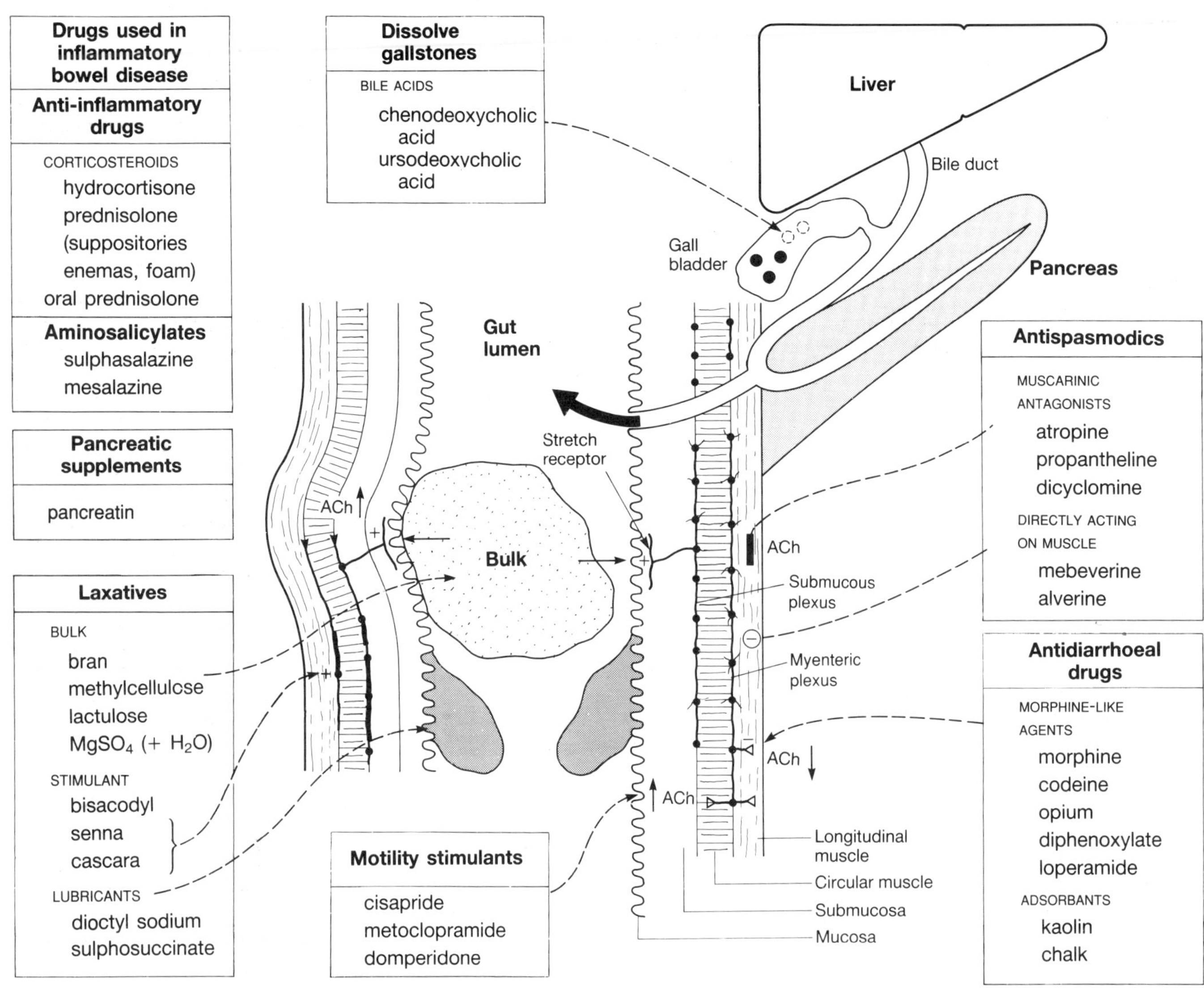

Muscular contractions of the gut and secretion of acid and enzymes are under autonomic control. The enteric part of the autonomic nervous system consists of ganglionated plexuses (⊣—⊢) with complex interconnections supplying the smooth muscle, mucosa and blood vessels. The ganglia (⋏) (parasympathetic) receive extrinsic excitatory fibres from the vagus and inhibitory sympathetic fibres.

Cholinomimetic drugs (e.g. *carbachol*, *neostigmine*) increase motility and may cause colic and diarrhoea. They are very occasionally used in the treatment of paralytic ileus (Chapter 8). More useful **motility stimulants** (bottom middle) facilitate acetylcholine release from the myenteric plexus and are used in the treatment of oesophageal reflux and gastric stasis. **Laxatives** (bottom left) are drugs used to increase the motility of the gut and encourage defaecation. *Bulk* (▒) laxatives stimulate stretch receptors in the mucosa. *Stimulant laxatives* stimulate the myenteric plexus and some drugs act as *lubricants* (▓).

Muscarinic antagonists and drugs that directly relax smooth muscle (top right) reduce gastrointestinal motility and are used to reduce spasm in irritable bowel syndrome (**antispasmodics**). **Antidiarrhoeal drugs** (bottom right) include antimotility drugs, but replacement of water and electrolyte loss is generally more important than drug treatment, especially in infants and in infectious diarrhoea.

Anti-inflammatory corticosteroids and aminosalicylates (top left) are used in ulcerative colitis and Crohn's disease. To reduce the need for systemic steroids it is usual to add *azathioprine*, an immunosuppressant (Chapter 40).

In the duodenum, bile from the liver (top right) and pancreatic juice from the pancreas (right □) enters (⬅) usually through a common opening which is restricted by the sphincter of Oddi. **Bile acids** (top middle) are sometimes used to dissolve cholesterol gallstones (●). **Pancreatic supplements** (left middle) are given orally when the secretion of pancreatic juice is absent or reduced.

MOTILITY STIMULANTS

Metoclopramide is a dopamine antagonist and by blocking central dopamine receptors in the chemoreceptor trigger zone it produces an antinausea/antiemetic action (see also Chapter 26). The drug also increases contractions in the stomach and enhances the tone of the lower oesophageal sphincter, actions that combine to speed the transit of contents from the stomach. The prokinetic actions of metoclopramide are blocked by atropine, suggesting that they result from the facilitation of acetylcholine release from the myenteric plexus rather than by dopamine antagonism. *Domperidone* has similar actions but is less likely to enter the brain (see Chapter 25). *Cisapride* also increases gut motility by facilitating acetylcholine release but it does not have dopamine antagonist activity and is not an antiemetic.

LAXATIVES

Constipation is characterized by abdominal discomfort, loss of appetite and malaise resulting from insufficient frequency of defaecation resulting in abnormally hard and dry faeces. The frequency and volume of defaecation are best regulated by diet, but drugs may be needed for specific purposes (e.g. before surgery of the colon or rectum).

Bulk laxatives increase the volume of the intestinal contents stimulating peristalsis. They include indigestible polysaccharides such as cellulose (bran), methylcellulose and lactulose (a semi-synthetic disaccharide) and *osmotic agents*, which are salts containing poorly absorbed ions (e.g. $MgSO_4$, Epsom salts).

Stimulant laxatives increase motility by acting on the mucosa or nerve plexuses, which may be damaged by prolonged drug use. They often cause abdominal cramp. *Anthraquinones* are released from precursor glycosides present in senna and cascara. They stimulate the myenteric plexus. Bisacodyl may act by stimulating sensory nerve endings.

Lubricants promote defaecation by softening (e.g. dioctyl sodium sulphosuccinate) and/or lubricating (e.g. liquid paraffin) faeces and assisting evacuation. Chronic use of liquid paraffin may impair absorption of the fat-soluble vitamins A and D and cause paraffinomas.

ANTIDIARRHOEAL DRUGS

Infectious diarrhoea is a very common cause of illness which results in a high mortality in developing countries. Bacterial pathogens cause the most severe forms of infectious diarrhoea, but more often diarrhoea is caused by a viral infection.

Antimotility drugs are widely used to provide symptomatic relief in mild to moderate forms of acute diarrhoea. Opioids such as *morphine*, *diphenoxylate*, and *codeine* activate μ-receptors on myenteric neurones and cause hyperpolarization by increasing their potassium conductance. This inhibits acetylcholine release from the myenteric plexus and reduces bowel motility. *Loperamide* is the most appropriate opioid for local effects on the gut because it does not easily penetrate to the brain. Hence, it has few central actions and is unlikely to cause dependence.

Adsorbants such as *kaolin*, either alone or with other drugs, are popular remedies for diarrhoeal illnesses, but there is little evidence that they do any good.

Rehydration therapy. Oral solutions containing electrolytes and glucose are given to correct the severe dehydration that can be caused by infection with toxigenic organisms.

Antibiotics are useful only in certain specific infections, e.g. cholera and severe bacillary dysentry, which are treated with tetracycline. The quinolones (Chapter 35) are more recent agents that seem to be effective against most important diarrhoeal pathogens.

DRUGS USED IN INFLAMMATORY BOWEL DISEASE

Inflammatory bowel disease is divided into two types: (1) *Crohn's disease*, which can affect the entire gut; and (2) *ulcerative colitis*, which affects only the large bowel. Local or systemic anti-inflammatory **corticosteroids**, e.g. *prednisolone* (Chapter 31) are the main drugs used for acute attacks, but their serious adverse effects make them unsuitable for maintenance treatment. **Aminosalicylates** reduce the symptoms in mild disease and maintenance treatment reduces the relapse rates of patients in remission. *Sulphasalazine* is a combination of 5-aminosalicylic acid with a sulphonamide. The molecule is cleaved in the colon by bacteria, releasing 5-aminosalicylic acid, which is the active moiety, and sulphapyridine, which is absorbed and may produce the adverse effects characteristic of sulphonamides (e.g. nausea, rashes, blood disorders) (see Chapter 35). Newer, less toxic drugs are *mesalazine*, which is 5-aminosalicylate in a preparation that releases the drug in the colon, and *olsalazine* (azodisalicylate) which consists of two molecules of 5-aminosalicylic acid joined by an azo bond, which is cleaved by bacteria in the colon. The mechanism of action of 5-aminosalicylate is unknown.

DRUGS USED TO DISSOLVE GALLSTONES

Bile contains cholesterol, phospholipids and bile salts, the latter being important in keeping cholesterol in solution. An increase in cholesterol concentration or a decrease in bile salts may result in the formation of cholesterol stones. If they give rise to symptoms, surgical removal is the usual form of treatment. However, small non-calcified stones may be dissolved by prolonged oral administration of the bile acids *chenodeoxycholic* or *ursodeoxycholic acid*, which decrease the cholesterol content of bile by inhibiting an enzyme involved in cholesterol formation. Chenodeoxycholic acid often causes diarrhoea and sometimes liver abnormalities.

PANCREATIC SUPPLEMENTS

Pancreatic juice contains important enzymes which break down proteins (trypsin, chymotrypsin), starch (amylase) and fats (lipase). In some diseases (e.g. chronic pancreatitis and cystic fibrosis) there is an absence or reduction in these enzymes. Patients with pancreatic insufficiency are given *pancreatin*, an extract of pancreas containing protease, lipase and amylase. Because the enzymes are inactivated by gastric acid, it is usual to give an H_2-receptor antagonist (e.g. *cimetidine*) beforehand. Newer enteric-coated preparations that deliver more of the enzymes to the duodenum are available.

14 Drugs acting on the kidney—diuretics

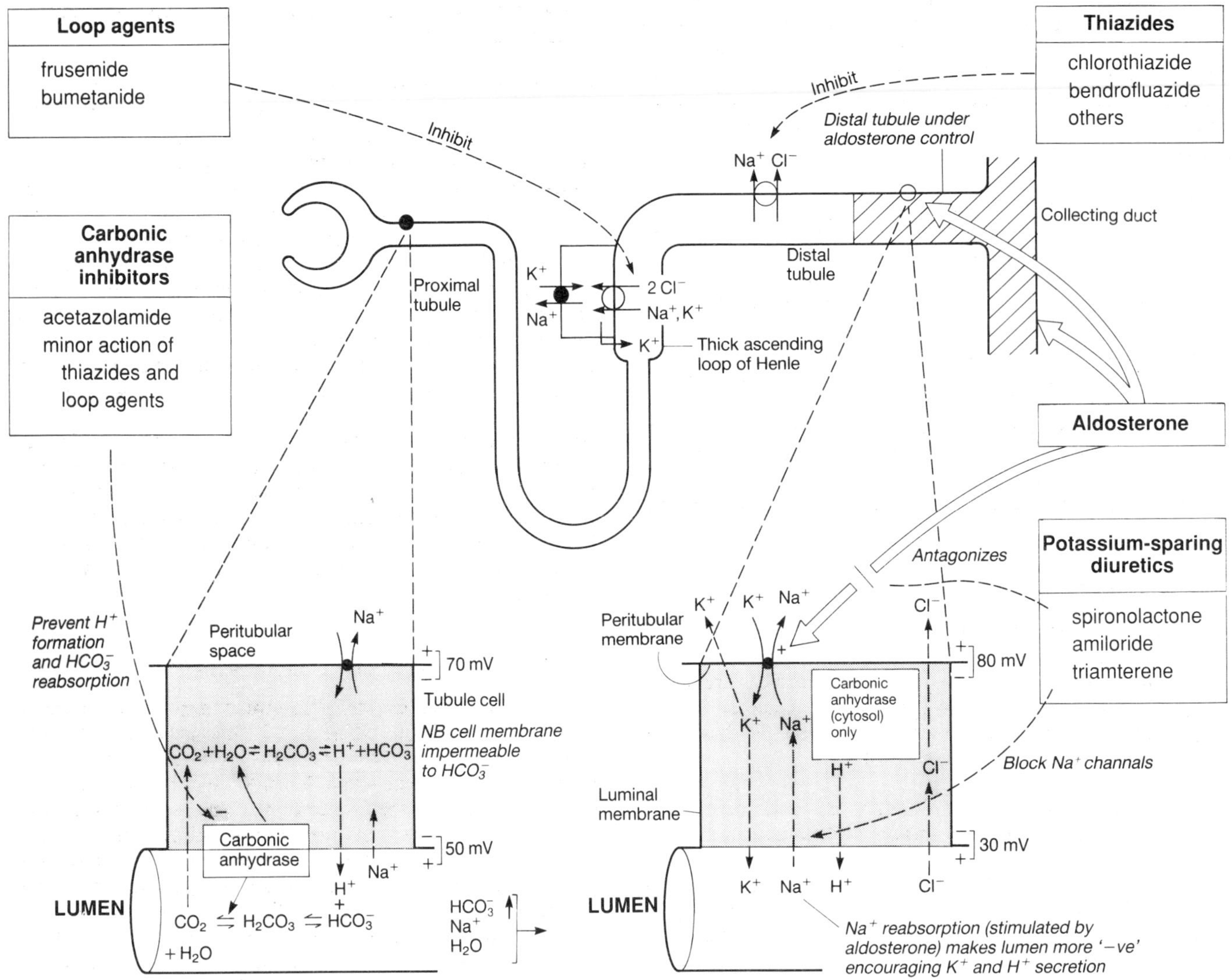

Diuretics are drugs that act on the kidney to increase urine flow. Most work by reducing the reabsorption of electrolytes by the tubules (top). The increased electrolyte excretion is accompanied by an increase in water excretion, necessary to maintain an osmotic balance. Diuretics are used to reduce oedema in *congestive heart failure*, some *renal diseases* and *hepatic cirrhosis*. Some diuretics, notably the thiazides, are widely used in the treatment of *hypertension*, but their long-term hypotensive action is not only related to their diuretic properties.

The **thiazides** and related compounds (top right) are safe, orally active, but relatively weak diuretics. More potent drugs are the **high ceiling** or **loop diuretics** (top left). These drugs have a very rapid onset, and fairly short duration of action. They are very powerful (hence the term 'high ceiling') and can cause serious electrolyte imbalances and dehydration. The thiazides, and especially the loop diuretics, increase potassium excretion and potassium supplements may be required to prevent hypokalaemia.

Some diuretics are '**potassium sparing**' (bottom right). They are weak when used alone, but they cause potassium retention, and are often given with thiazides or loop diuretics to prevent hypokalaemia.

Carbonic anhydrase inhibitors (bottom left figure) are weak diuretics and are rarely used for their diuretic action. **Osmotic diuretics** (e.g. *mannitol*) are compounds which are filtered but not reabsorbed. They are excreted with an osmotic equivalent of water and are sometimes used in forced diuresis to treat drug overdosage, in cerebral oedema, and to maintain a diuresis during surgery.

The kidney is one of the major routes of drug elimination, and impairment of renal function in old age or in renal disease can significantly decrease the elimination of drugs.

Aldosterone stimulates Na^+ reabsorption in the distal tubule and increases K^+ and H^+ secretion. It acts on cytoplasmic receptors (Chapter 31) and induces the synthesis of a protein, which either increases the availability of Na^+ entry sites in the luminal membrane or increases the activity of Na^+/K^+ ATPase in the peritubular membrane. Diuretics *increase* the Na^+ load in the distal tubule and, except for the potassium-sparing agents, this results in an *increased K^+ secretion* (and excretion). This effect is greater if plasma aldosterone levels are high; for example if vigorous diuretic therapy has depleted the body of Na^+ stores.

Carbonic anhydrase inhibitors depress bicarbonate reabsorption in the proximal tubule by inhibiting the catalysis of CO_2 hydration/dehydration reactions. Thus, the excretion of HCO_3^-, Na^+ and H_2O is increased. The loss of HCO_3^- causes a metabolic acidosis and, because H^+ ions are formed even without carbonic anhydrase, these drugs are quickly self-limiting. The increased Na^+ delivered to the distal nephron increases K^+ secretion, an effect made more severe by the lack of the normal competition for secretion by H^+ ions. *Acetazolamide* is used in glaucoma to reduce intraocular pressure, which it does by reducing the secretion of HCO_3^- and associated H_2O into the aqueous humour (Chapter 10). It is also used as a prophylactic agent for mountain (altitude) sickness.

THIAZIDES

Thiazides were developed from the carbonic anhydrase inhibitors. However, the diuretic activity of these drugs is not related to their effects on this enzyme. The thiazides are widely used in the treatment of mild heart failure (Chapter 18) and hypertension (Chapter 15), in which condition they have been shown to reduce the incidence of stroke.

Mechanism. Thiazides act mainly on the early segments of the *distal tubule*, where they *inhibit NaCl reabsorption*. The mechanism of this inhibition involves blockade of electroneutral cotransport of Na^+–Cl^- from the lumen into the tubular cells. Excretion of Cl^-, Na^+ and accompanying H_2O is increased. The increased Na^+ load in the distal tubule stimulates Na^+ exchange with K^+ and H^+, increasing their excretion and causing hypokalaemia and a metabolic alkalosis.

Adverse effects. These are important because thiazides may be taken for life. They may cause *weakness*, *impotence* and occasionally *skin rashes*. Serious allergic reactions (e.g. thrombocytopenia) are rare. More common are metabolic effects:
1 **Hypokalaemia** may precipitate cardiac arrhythmias, especially in patients on digitalis. This can be prevented by giving potassium supplements if necessary, or by combined therapy with a potassium-sparing diuretic.
2 **Uric acid** levels in the blood are often increased (hyperuricaemia) because thiazides are secreted by the organic acid secretory system in the tubules and compete for uric acid secretion. This may precipitate *gout*.
3 **Lipids.** Thiazides increase plasma cholesterol levels, at least during the first 6 months of administration. It is not certain whether prolonged treatment results in the blood lipids returning to normal and the significance (if any) of the effects of thiazides on cholesterol is uncertain.

LOOP DIURETICS

Loop diuretics can be given orally or, in emergencies, intravenously. They are used to reduce peripheral and pulmonary oedema in moderate and severe heart failure (Chapter 18). Unlike the thiazides they are effective in patients with diminished renal function.

Mechanism. Loop agents have a thiazide-like action on the early distal tubule, but much more importantly, they *inhibit NaCl reabsorption* in the *thick ascending loop of Henle*. This segment has a high capacity for absorbing NaCl and so drugs which act on this site produce a diuresis that is much greater than that of other diuretics. Loop diuretics act on the luminal membrane where they inhibit the cotransport of Na^+–K^+–$2Cl^-$. (The Na^+ is actively transported out of the cells into the interstitium by an Na^+/K^+ ATPase dependent pump in the basolateral membrane.) The specificity of the loop diuretics is due to their high local concentration in the renal tubules. However, at high doses, these drugs may induce changes in the electrolyte composition of the endolymph and cause deafness.

Adverse effects. Like the thiazides, the loop agents have hyperglycaemic, hyperuricaemic, hypotensive and hypokalaemic effects. Potassium loss may be considerable and, with regular use, potassium supplements are needed more often than with thiazides. Overenthusiastic use of loop diuretics (high doses, intravenous administration) can cause *deafness*, which may not be reversible.

POTASSIUM-SPARING DIURETICS

These diuretics act on the aldosterone responsive segments of the distal nephron, where K^+ homeostasis is controlled. *Aldosterone* stimulates Na^+ reabsorption, generating a negative potential in the lumen, which drives K^+ and H^+ ions into the lumen (and hence their excretion). The potassium-sparing diuretics reduce Na^+ reabsorption by either antagonizing aldosterone (spironolactone) or blocking Na^+ channels (amiloride, triamterene). This causes the electrical potential across the tubular epithelium to fall, reducing the driving force for K^+ secretion. The drugs may cause severe hyperkalaemia, especially in patients with renal impairment. Hyperkalaemia is also likely to occur if the patients are also taking inhibitors of angiotensin converting enzyme (e.g. captopril), because these drugs reduce aldosterone secretion.

Spironolactone competitively blocks the binding of aldosterone to its cytoplasmic receptor and so increases the excretion of Na^+ (Cl^- and H_2O) and decreases the 'electrically coupled' K^+ secretion. It is a weak diuretic, because only 2% of the total Na^+ reabsorption is under aldosterone control. Some metabolites of spironolactone have been shown to be carcinogenic in rats and the drug is now only used in liver disease with ascites and Conn's syndrome (primary hyperaldosteronism).

Amiloride and triamterene decrease the luminal membrane Na^+ permeability in the distal nephron by combining with Na^+ channels and blocking them on a 1:1 basis. This increases Na^+ (Cl^- and H_2O) excretion and decreases K^+ excretion.

15 Drugs used in hypertension

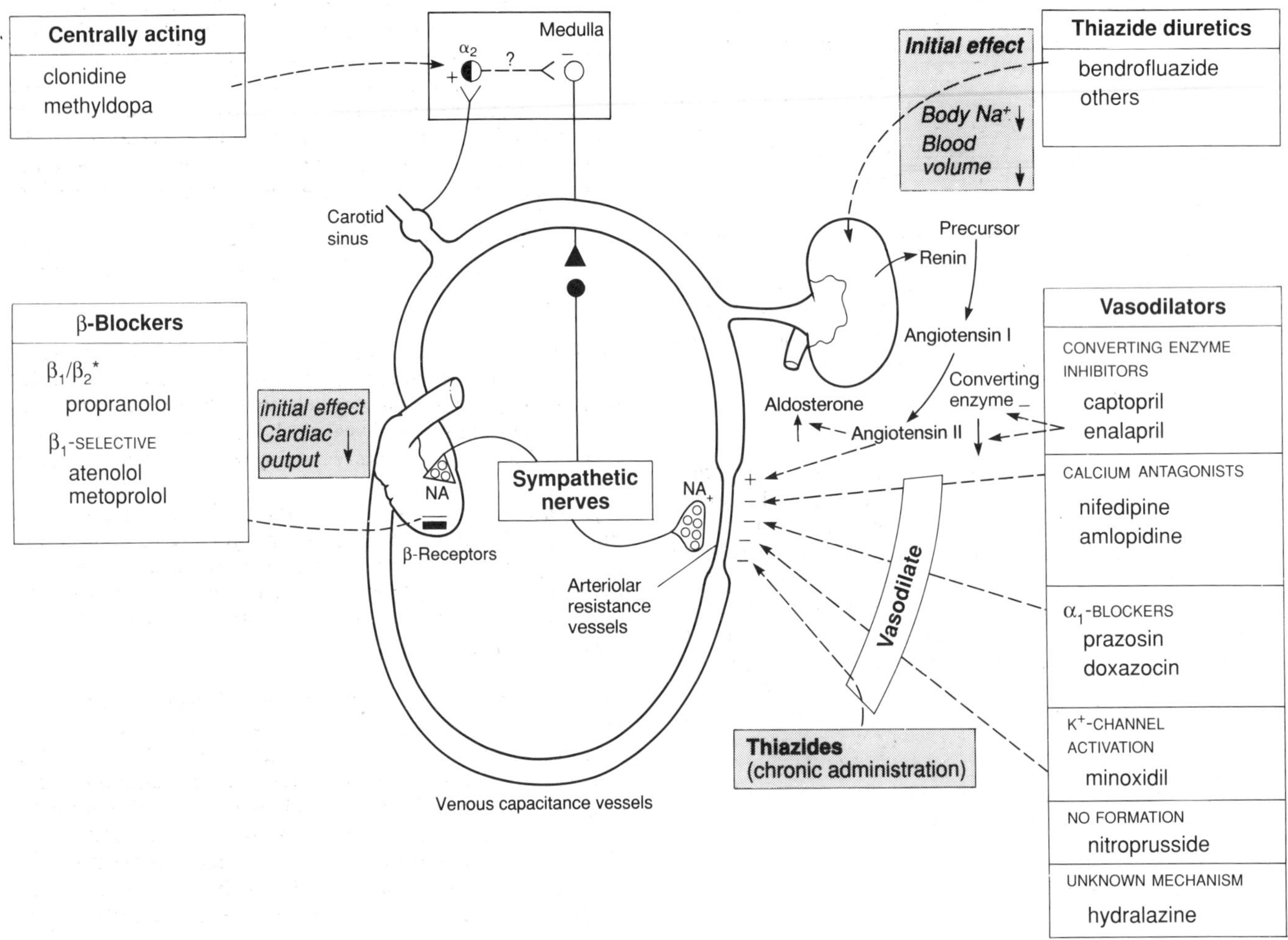

Hypertension is difficult to define precisely, but it is generally accepted that therapy is indicated if the diastolic pressure regularly exceeds 100 mmHg. Most patients have primary (essential) hypertension for which there is no obvious cause, but a small percentage have hypertension secondary to renal or endocrine disease.

It is important to lower the blood pressure of hypertensives, because high blood pressure is associated with a decreased life expectancy and serious complications, including congestive heart failure, cerebral haemorrhage, renal failure and retinopathy. Reduction of blood pressure reduces the mortality and morbidity of hypertensives (except perhaps the elderly), but treatment, once started, is usually required for life and should not be undertaken lightly. Smoking should be discouraged strongly because it is an independent and supra-additive risk factor for vascular disease.

In some mild hypertensives, weight reduction, if appropriate, and moderate reduction in salt consumption may be sufficient, but usually drug treatment is required. The **β-adrenoceptor antagonists** (β-blockers, centre left) and the **thiazide diuretics** (top right) are presently the first-line drugs in the treatment of hypertension. In neither case is their mode of action clear. Several groups of drugs, by different mechanisms, reduce blood pressure by decreasing vasoconstrictor tone and hence peripheral resistance. The most important of these are the angiotensin converting enzyme inhibitors (**ACE inhibitors**) (middle right), which decrease circulating angiotensin II (a vasoconstrictor), and the **calcium antagonists** (middle right) which block the entry of calcium into vascular smooth muscle cells. Other vasodilators (bottom right) have been largely superseded by the ACE inhibitors and calcium antagonists, although there is some interest in selective **α_1-adrenoceptor antagonists**, mainly because it is claimed that they have 'favourable' effects on blood lipids. **Centrally acting drugs** (top left) decrease sympathetic outflow by stimulating central α_2-adrenoceptors but are little used currently, because of their adverse effects.

Mild to moderate hypertension can often be controlled by a single drug, but if this fails the traditional approach is to combine two drugs (e.g. diuretic and β-blocker) and add a third if necessary (e.g. a peripheral vasodilator).

THIAZIDE DIURETICS

The mechanism by which diuretics reduce arterial blood pressure is not known. Initially, the blood pressure falls because of a decrease in blood volume, venous return and cardiac output. Gradually, the cardiac output returns to normal, but the hypotensive effect remains because the peripheral resistance has, in the meantime, decreased. Diuretics have no direct effect on vascular smooth muscle and the vasodilatation they cause seems to be associated with a small but persistent reduction in body Na^+. One possible mechanism is that a fall in smooth muscle Na^+ causes a secondary reduction in intracellular Ca^{2+} so that the muscle becomes less responsive. Thiazide diuretics may cause *hypokalaemia, diabetes mellitus, gout* and change the blood lipids in an 'atherogenic' way (see also Chapter 14). In addition to these metabolic side-effects, recent studies have emphasized that 'trivial' side-effects such as impotence, diarrhoea, tinnitus and loss of libido are more common with thiazide usage than with β-blockers.

β-ADRENOCEPTOR ANTAGONISTS

β-Blockers initially produce a fall in blood pressure by decreasing the cardiac output. With continued treatment, the cardiac output returns to normal but the blood pressure remains low, because, by an unknown mechanism, the peripheral vascular resistance is 'reset' at a lower level (individual drugs are discussed in Chapter 9). Disadvantages of β-blockade are the common adverse effects such as cold hands, fatigue and the less common, but serious adverse effects, such as the *provocation* of *asthma, heart failure* or *conductance block*. β-Blockers also tend to raise serum triglyceride and decrease HDL-cholesterol levels. All the β-blockers lower blood pressure but at least some of the side-effects can be reduced by using cardio-selective hydrophilic drugs (i.e. those without liver metabolism or brain penetration) such as atenolol.

VASODILATOR DRUGS

ACE inhibitors. Angiotensin II is a powerful circulating vasoconstrictor and inhibition of its synthesis in hypertensive subjects results in a fall in peripheral resistance and a lowering of blood pressure. ACE inhibitors do not impair cardiovascular reflexes and are devoid of many of the adverse effects of the diuretics and β-blockers. Rare but serious adverse effects of ACE inhibitors include angio-oedema, proteinuria and neutropenia. The first dose may cause a very steep fall in blood pressure, e.g. in patients on diuretics (because they are Na^+ depleted). Less serious side-effects include a dry cough, skin rashes and loss of sense of smell. ACE inhibitors may cause renal failure in patients with bilateral renal artery stenosis, because in this condition angiotensin II is apparently required to constrict glomerular arterioles and maintain adequate glomerular filtration. Inhibition of angiotensin II formation reduces, but does not seriously impair, aldosterone secretion and excessive K^+ retention only occurs in patients taking potassium-supplements or potassium-sparing diuretics (aldosterone increases Na^+ reabsorption and K^+ excretion, Chapter 14).

Calcium antagonists. The tone of vascular smooth muscle is determined by the cytosolic Ca^{2+} concentration. This is increased by α_1-adrenoceptor activation (resulting from sympathetic tone) which triggers Ca^{2+} release from the sarcoplasmic reticulum via the second-messenger inositol trisphosphate (Chapter 1). There also seem to be receptor-operated cation channels, about which little is known. Nevertheless they are important because the entry of cations through them depolarizes the cell, opening voltage dependent (L-type) Ca^{2+} channels which causes additional Ca^{2+} to enter the cell. The calcium antagonists bind to the L-type channels and by blocking the entry of Ca^{2+} into the cell they cause relaxation of the arteriolar smooth muscle. This reduces the peripheral resistance and results in a fall in blood pressure. The efficacy of calcium antagonists is similar to that of the thiazides and β-blockers. Their most common side-effects are due to excessive vasodilatation and include dizziness, hypotension, flushing and ankle oedema.

α-Adrenoceptor antagonists. *Prazosin* and the longer acting *doxazosin* cause vasodilatation by selectively blocking vascular α_1-adrenoceptors. Unlike non-selective α-blockers, these drugs are not likely to cause tachycardia, but they may cause postural hypotension. Severe hypotension may occur after the first dose.

Hydralazine is used in combination with a β-blocker and diuretic. Side-effects include reflex tachycardia which may provoke angina, headaches and fluid retention (due to secondary hyperaldosteronism). In slow acetylators particularly, hydralazine may induce a *lupus syndrome* resulting in fever, arthralgia, malaise and hepatitis.

Minoxidil (active metabolite, minoxidil NO sulphate) is a potent vasodilator which causes severe fluid retention and oedema. However, when given with a β-blocker and loop diuretic, it is effective in severe hypertension resistant to other drug combinations. Minoxidil sulphate opens ATP-sensitive K^+ channels in vascular smooth muscle cells, causing hyperpolarization and relaxation. These K^+ channels are normally kept closed by intracellular ATP, which is apparently antagonized by minoxidil sulphate (cf. oral antidiabetic drugs, Chapter 34).

CENTRALLY ACTING DRUGS

Methyldopa is converted in adrenergic nerve endings to the false transmitter, α-methylnoradrenaline, which stimulates α_2-receptors in the medulla and reduces sympathetic outflow. Postural hypotension may occur, and in 20% of patients it causes a positive antiglobulin (Coomb's) test and, rarely, haemolytic anaemia. **Clonidine** causes rebound hypertension if the drug is suddenly withdrawn.

ACUTE SEVERE HYPERTENSION

In hypertensive crisis, drugs may be given by intravenous infusion (e.g. **hydralazine** in hypertension associated with eclampsia of pregnancy; **nitroprusside** in malignant hypertension with encephalopathy). However, intravenous drugs are rarely necessary, and the trend is to use oral agents whenever possible. Nitroprusside decomposes in the blood to release nitric oxide (NO), an unstable compound that causes vasodilatation (see Chapter 16 for mechanism).

16 Drugs used in angina

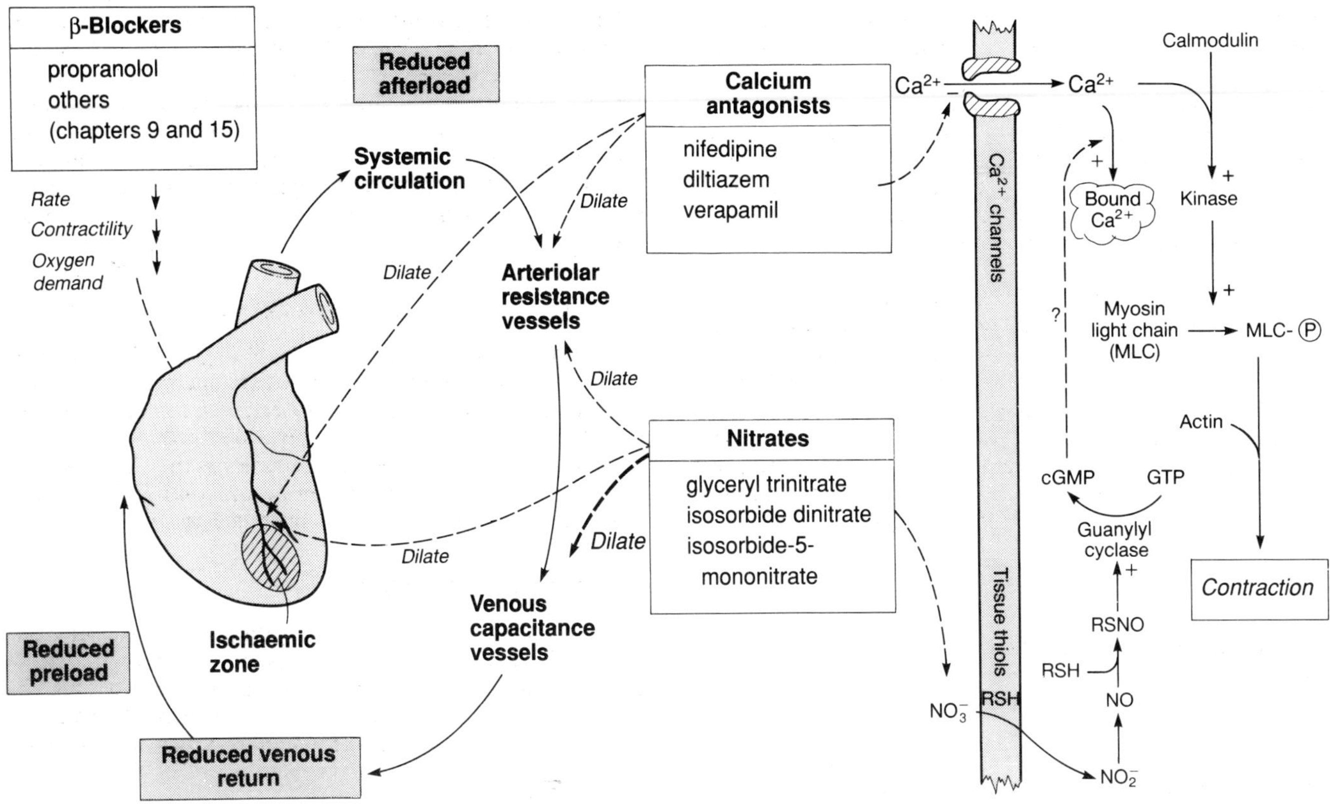

The coronary arteries supply blood to the heart. With increasing age, atheromatous plaques progressively narrow the arteries, and the obstruction to blood flow may eventually become so severe that when exercise increases the oxygen consumption of the heart, not enough blood can pass through the arteries to supply it. The ischaemic muscle then produces the characteristic pain of angina, probably because waste products released during muscle contraction accumulate in the poorly perfused tissue.

The basic aim of drug treatment in angina is to reduce the work of the heart and hence its oxygen demand. The **nitrates** (lower-middle) are the first-line drugs. Their main effect is to cause peripheral vasodilatation, especially in the veins, by an action on the vascular smooth muscle that involves the formation of nitric oxide (NO) and an increase in intracellular cGMP (right figure). The resulting pooling of blood in the capacitance vessels (veins) reduces venous return and the ventricular volume is decreased. Reduction in the distension of the heart wall decreases oxygen demand and the pain is quickly relieved.

Sublingual *glyceryl trinitrate* is used to treat acute anginal attacks. If this is ineffective then combined therapy is required in which **β-adrenoceptor blockers** (top left) or **calcium antagonists** (middle top) are taken in addition to glyceryl trinitrate, which is retained for acute attacks.

β-Adrenoceptor blockers depress myocardial contractility and reduce the heart rate. In addition to these effects, which reduce the oxygen demand, β-blockers may also increase the perfusion of the ischaemic area, because the decrease in heart rate increases the duration of diastole and hence the time available for coronary blood flow.

β-Blockers are the standard drugs used in angina, but they have many side-effects and contraindications (Chapter 15). Hence the **calcium antagonists**, which have fewer serious side-effects are increasingly used in place of β-blockers as an adjunct to short-acting nitrates. Calcium antagonists have actions on the heart, but they relieve angina mainly by causing peripheral arteriolar dilatation and afterload reduction. They are useful if there is some degree of coronary artery spasm.

Preload and afterload. The force of contraction of cardiac muscle, and hence its oxygen demand, is dependent on its preloading and afterloading. The preload is the degree to which the myocardium is stretched before it contracts and depends on the venous return. The afterload is the resistance against which the blood is expelled. Reduction of either the preload or afterload will reduce the work of the heart and hence its oxygen demand.

Angina pectoris is a description of a typical set of symptoms related to myocardial ischaemia and usually due to underlying atheromatous narrowing of the coronary arteries. These symptoms include a feeling of tightness in the chest, usually retrosternal and often radiating to the arms, precipitated by exercise and relieved by rest and nitrates.

Stable and unstable angina. In 'stable' angina there is little change in the pain or the frequency of the attacks. When, however, the symptoms are of sudden or recent onset, or are progressing in severity or frequency, occuring at lesser levels of exertion or at rest, the term 'unstable angina' may be applied. Unstable angina has a different pathology and probably results from fissuring of an atheromatous plaque with subsequent platelet aggregation. In these patients, antiplatelet treatment with aspirin in addition to antianginal drugs is very effective.

NITRATES

Short-acting nitrates. Sublingual glyceryl trinitrate acts for about 30 minutes. It is more useful in preventing attacks than in stopping them once they have begun.

Long-acting nitrates are more stable and may be effective for several hours, depending on the drug and preparation used (sublingual, oral, transdermal, oral sustained-release). Isosorbide dinitrate is widely used, but it is rapidly metabolized by the liver. The use of isosorbide-5-mononitrate, which is the main active metabolite of the dinitrate, avoids the variable absorption and unpredictable first-pass metabolism of the dinitrate. The prophylactic value of long-acting nitrates is uncertain, but they are a rational choice for the acute treatment of unstable angina.

Adverse effects. The arterial dilatation produced by the nitrates causes facial flushing and headaches, which frequently limit the dose. More serious side-effects are hypotension and fainting. Reflex tachycardia often occurs, but this is prevented by combined therapy with β-blockers. Prolonged high dosage may cause methaemoglobinaemia due to oxidation of haemoglobin.

Mechanism of action. Metabolism of the drugs first releases nitrite ions (NO_2^-), a process that requires tissue thiols. Within the cell, NO_2^- is converted first to nitric oxide (NO) and then to a *S*-nitrosothiol derivative by reaction with thiols. The *S*-nitrosothiol derivative activates guanylyl cyclase, causing an increase in the intracellular concentration of guanosine 3′,5′-monophosphate (cyclic GMP) in the vascular smooth muscle cells. Precisely how the cGMP causes relaxation is not clear, but it eventually results in the dephosphorylation of the myosin light chain (MLC) possibly by decreasing the concentration of free Ca^{2+} ions in the cytosol. (Phosphorylation of MLC initiates the interaction of myosin with actin and muscle contraction.)

Tolerance may occur to nitrates. For example, chronic pentaerthrytol tetranitrate has been shown to produce tolerance to sublingual glyceryl trinitrate and moderate doses of oral isosorbide dinitrate four times a day produces tolerance with loss of the antianginal effect. However, twice daily dosing of isosorbide dinitrate at 0800 and 1300 hours does not produce tolerance, presumably because the overnight rest allows tissue sensitivity to return by the next day. Tolerance to nitrates maybe caused by depletion of sulphydryl group donors, since tolerance to nitrates both *in vitro* and *in vivo* is reversed by *N*-acetylcysteine.

β-ADRENOCEPTOR ANTAGONISTS

β-Blockers are used for prophylaxis of angina. The choice of drug may be important. *Intrinsic activity* might be a *disadvantage* in angina, and the cardioselective β-blockers such as *atenolol* and *metoprolol* are probably the drugs of choice. All β-blockers are best avoided in asthmatics as they may precipitate bronchospasm. The *adverse effects* and contraindications of β-blockers should be reviewed (Chapters 9 and 15).

CALCIUM ANTAGONISTS

These drugs are widely used in the treatment of angina and have fewer serious side-effects than β-blockers. *Diltiazem* has fewest side-effects and only a slight negative inotropic effect, but is less potent than *nifedipine*. *Verapamil* is the drug of choice in patients who have supraventricular arrhythmias in addition to angina.

Prinzmetal's angina. This uncommon 'variant' form of angina is less convincingly associated with exercise, and coronary angiography may reveal coronary artery spasm which may be at least partially responsible for the pain. β-Blockers may make things worse by producing unopposed α-adrenergic tone in the coronary arteries. *Nitrates* and *calcium antagonists* are effective in this form of angina, because of their direct vasodilator action on the coronary arteries.

Tobacco smoking. Smoking reduces coronary blood flow and the nicotine-induced rise in heart rate and blood pressure increases the oxygen demand of the heart. In addition, the formation of carboxyhaemoglobin reduces the oxygen carrying capacity of the blood. Some patients improve remarkably on giving up smoking.

Coronary artery bypass or **percutaneous transarterial coronary angioplasty (PTCA)**, may be indicated in patients not responding to drugs. In bypass operations, a segment of saphenous vein or internal mammary artery is inserted between the aorta and a point beyond the stenosis of the affected coronary artery. Angina is relieved or improved in 90% of patients, but returns in 50% within 7 years. Mortality is decreased in some pathological conditions (e.g. left main coronary artery disease). In PTCA a balloon catheter is used to split and compress the atheromatous plaque.

17 Antiarrhythmic drugs

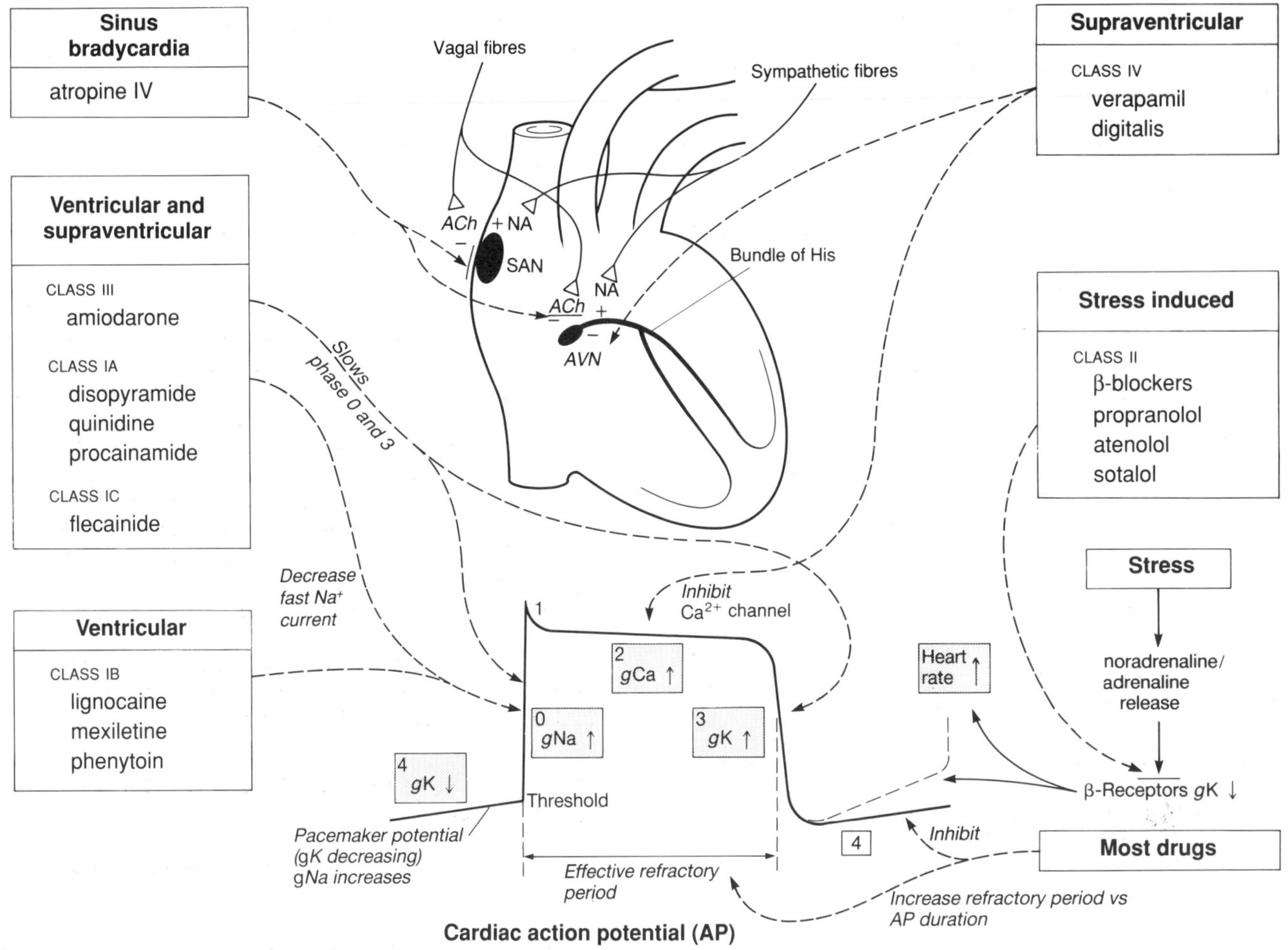

Cardiac action potential (AP)

The rhythm of the heart is normally determined by **pacemaker** cells in the sinoatrial node (SAN, top), but it can be disturbed in a variety of ways, producing anything from occasional discomfort to the symptoms of heart failure. Arrhythmias can occur in the apparently healthy heart, but serious ones are usually associated with heart disease. The rhythm of the heart is affected by both **acetylcholine** (ACh) and **noradrenaline** (NA), released from parasympathetic and sympathetic nerves respectively (upper figure).

Supraventricular arrhythmias arise in the atrial myocardium or atrioventricular node (AVN), whilst ventricular arrhythmias originate in the ventricles. Arrhythmias may be caused by an **ectopic focus**, which starts firing at a higher rate than the normal pacemaker (SAN). More commonly, a **re-entry** mechanism is involved, where action potentials, delayed for some pathological reason, re-invade nearby muscle fibres which, being no longer refractory, again depolarize, establishing a loop of depolarization (circus movement).

Most antiarrhythmic drugs have local anaesthetic activity (i.e. block voltage-dependent Na^+ channels), or are calcium antagonists. These actions decrease the automaticity of pacemaker cells and increase the effective refractory period of atrial, ventricular and Purkinje fibres.

Antiarrhythmic agents can be classified into: (1) those which are effective in **supraventricular arrhythmias** (top right); (2) those effective in **ventricular arrhythmias** (bottom left); and (3) those effective on **both types** (middle left). Arrhythmias associated with stress conditions in which there is an increase in adrenergic activity (emotion, excitement, thyrotoxicosis, myocardial infarction) may be treated with β-blockers (bottom right). An arrhythmia common after acute myocardial infarction is sinus bradycardia, which can be treated with intravenous atropine if the cardiac output is lowered (top left). Antiarrhythmics have also been classified on the basis of their electrophysiological effects on Purkinje fibres (roman numerals). The effects of antiarrhythmic agents on the **cardiac action potential** are shown in the lower figure, but it is not usually known how these actions relate to the drugs' therapeutic effects. Sometimes drugs can be avoided by **alternative treatment** (e.g. DC shock, pacemakers).

CARDIAC ACTION POTENTIAL

Cardiac cells have two depolarizing currents, a fast Na^+ current and a slower Ca^{2+} current. In the SAN and AVN there is only a Ca^{2+} current and because pure 'Ca^{2+} spikes' conduct very slowly, there is a delay between atrial and ventricular contraction. The long refractory period of cardiac fibres normally protects them from re-excitation during a heart beat.

PACEMAKER CELLS

In the SAN and AVN, pacemaker cells possess a K^+ conductance, which gradually decreases, resulting in a depolarization drift. When the depolarization reaches threshold, an action potential is initiated. The slope of the pacemaker potentials in the SAN is greater than in the AVN and so the SAN normally determines the heart rate (sinus rhythm). The pacemaker and conducting cells receive autonomic innervation.

Acetylcholine. Vagal fibres release acetylcholine onto muscarinic receptors, the activation of which increases the K^+ conductance (gK) and decreases the slope of the pacemaker potential. Thus, the threshold for firing is reached later and the heart beat slows. Conductance in the bundle of His is also slowed. Antiarrhythmic drugs with atropine-like actions (e.g. disopyramide, quinidine) block vagal influence on the AVN and facilitate atrio–ventricular (A–V) conduction. In atrial flutter/fibrillation, this may result in dangerously increased ventricular rates, and so digitalis is given first to increase the A–V block.

Noradrenaline. Sympathetic fibres release noradrenaline onto β_1-receptors in the pacemaker tissues and myocardium. Noradrenaline decreases gK so threshold is reached earlier and the heart rate increases (positive chronotropic effect). Noradrenaline also increases the force of contraction by increasing gCa during the plateau phase (positive inotropic effect).

DRUGS EFFECTIVE IN VENTRICULAR AND SUPRAVENTRICULAR ARRHYTHMIAS

Class IA agents act by blocking (open) voltage-dependent Na^+ channels. They are essentially cardiac depressants, and act on the *atrial* and *ventricular muscle cells*, the *Purkinje fibres* and the *AV node*. They: (1) decrease the automaticity of the heart by slowing phase 4 of the cardiac action potential and by raising the threshold of phase 0; and (2) slow phase 0 and lengthen the effective refractory period.

Disopyramide is used orally to prevent ventricular arrhythmias and recurrent supraventricular arrhythmias (usually with digitalis). Disopyramide has as negative inotropic action and may cause hypotension (especially intravenously) and aggrevate cardiac failure. Other-side effects include anticholinergic effects, nausea and vomiting.

Quinidine is effective in the treatment of both supraventricular and ventricular arrhythmias, but its use is limited by potentially dangerous cardiac and frequent non-cardiac side-effects. Sustained-release tablets are used in the treatment of ventricular arrhythmias resistant to other drug treatment. Side-effects include anticholinergic effects, nausea, vomiting, diarrhoea and arrhythmias.

Procainamide has similar actions to quinidine but is not anticholinergic. Procainamide is little used now, because with chronic treatment 5–15% of patients develop a Lupus-like syndrome.

Class III agents act by slowing repolarization (phase 3) and prolong the duration of action potentials.

Amiodarone prolongs the effective refractory period, especially of Purkinje fibres and ventricular muscle cells. It is effective against many arrhythmias, but its use is restricted to patients in whom other drugs are ineffective, because it may cause serious adverse effects. These include photosensitivity (patients turn blue when exposed to sun), irreversible liver damage, thyroid disorders, neuropathy and pulmonary alveolitis.

Sotalol is a β-adrenoceptor antagonist with additional Class III activity. It is much safer than amiodarone but has the usual side-effects of β-blockers (Chapter 15).

DRUGS USED IN VENTRICULAR ARRHYTHMIAS

Class IB agents act by blocking (inactivated) voltage-dependent Na^+ channels.

Lignocaine given intravenously, is the first-line drug in the treatment of ventricular arrhythmias after acute myocardial infarction and cardiac surgery (it is inactive orally). Unlike Class IA drugs, lignocaine has few side-effects, although at high plasma concentrations it may cause drowsiness, agitation and, rarely, convulsions. In contrast to IA agents, which block open Na^+ channels, lignocaine blocks mainly inactivated Na^+ channels. In normal cardiac tissue, lignocaine has little effect because the Na^+ channels recover during diastole. However, in ischaemic areas, where anoxia causes depolarization and arrhythmogenic activity, many Na^+ channels are inactivated and therefore susceptible to lignocaine.

Mexiletine has similar actions as lignocaine. It can be given intravenously or orally but causes more cardiovascular and central adverse effects than lignocaine.

DRUGS EFFECTIVE IN SUPRAVENTRICULAR ARRHYTHMIAS

Class IV agents act by blocking Ca^{2+} channels (mainly L channels).

Verapamil has particularly powerful effects on the AVN, where conduction is entirely dependent on calcium spikes. Verapamil is effective in supraventricular arrhythmias, such as paroxysmal supraventricular tachycardia. Verapamil has a negative inotropic effect and may worsen cardiac failure. Intravenous combinations of β-blockers and verapamil may be fatal.

Digitalis (Chapter 18) slows conduction and prolongs the refractory period in the AVN and bundle of His. It is used in atrial fibrillation, which it does not stop, but it slows and strengthens the ventricular beat, mainly by reducing the frequency at which impulses pass along the conducting tissue.

ALTERNATIVES TO DRUGS

Pacemakers are required for complete heart block, and are sometimes used in tachyarrhythmias. When the left atrial size is normal, direct current shock causes reversion to sinus rhythm in most patients with atrial fibrillation, but about 60% relapse within 1 year despite maintenance treatment with disopyramide. Surgical ablation of the ectopic focus or bundle of His is a successful method of controlling supraventricular arrhythmias. A new and much safer method is ablation of the focus or bundle via electrodes on an intracardiac catheter (endocavity ablation). Since AV-block is produced, a permanent pacemaker is required.

18 Drugs used in heart failure

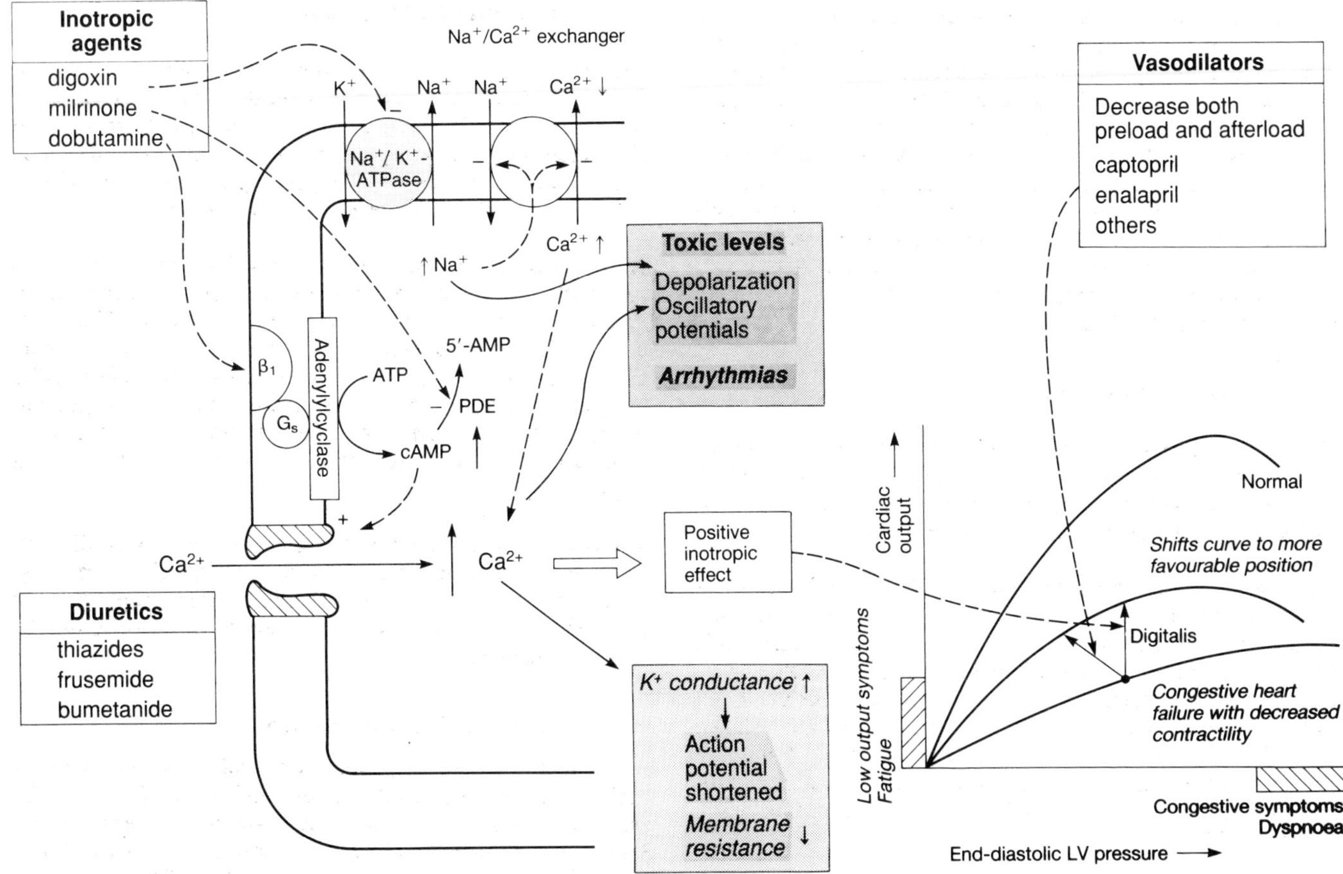

Heart failure exists when the cardiac output is insufficient to adequately perfuse the tissues. This leads to a variety of symptoms, e.g. fatigue, oedema and breathlessness. *Congestive heart failure* is usually taken to mean combined right and left heart failure, producing both pulmonary congestion and peripheral oedema. Common causes of heart failure include hypertension and coronary heart disease. The low cardiac output in heart failure results in increased sympathetic nervous activity which stimulates the rate and force of the heart beat and maintains the blood pressure by increasing the vascular resistance. The resulting increase in afterload further depresses cardiac output. Reduced renal blood flow results in *renin secretion* and increased plasma *angiotensin* and *aldosterone* levels. Sodium and water retention increase the blood volume, increasing the preload and the likelihood of oedema formation.

Traditionally, treatment of heart failure has usually started with **diuretics** (bottom left) (Chapter 14), which increase the excretion of sodium and water, and by reducing the circulatory volume, decrease the preload and oedema. However, treatment is changing and **vasodilators** (top right) are now often used first. *Angiotensin converting enzyme (ACE) inhibitors* reduce the load on the heart (right figure) and recent clinical trials have shown that they decrease symptoms and prolong life in congestive heart failure. If heart failure is so severe that a combination of diuretic and ACE inhibitor fails to provide an adequate response then an **inotropic drug** (top left) may be added. Inotropic drugs virtually all increase the force of cardiac muscle contraction by increasing the rise in cytosolic calcium that occurs with each action potential (left figure). Thus, both β-adrenoceptor agonists (e.g. *dobutamine*) and phosphodiesterase inhibitors (e.g. *milrinone*) increase the influx of Ca^{2+} via an increase in cAMP levels (left figure) whilst *digoxin* increases intracellular calcium indirectly, by inhibiting membrane Na^+/K^+ ATPase (◯). Inotropic drugs all tend to cause arrhythmias because excessive cytosolic calcium can trigger arrhythmogenic membrane currents. For this reason, there is considerable interest in investigational drugs called **calcium sensitizers** which increase the affinity of troponin C for calcium and so cause more force to be generated for a given amount of cytoplasmic calcium.

VASODILATOR DRUGS

Venous dilatation reduces the filling pressure (preload) and arteriolar dilatation lowers the resistance against which the heart has to pump (the afterload). The reduction in vascular tone decreases the work and oxygen demand of the failing heart. ACE inhibitors (e.g. **captopril**, **enalapril**) (see also Chapter 15) may be the most appropriate vasodilators in heart failure, because they lower both the arterial and venous resistance by preventing the increase in (vasoconstrictor) angiotensin II often present in heart failure. The cardiac output increases (diagonal arrow, right figure) and because the renovascular resistance falls, there is an increase in renal blood flow. This latter effect, together with reduced aldosterone release (angiotensin II is a stimulus for aldosterone release) increases Na^+ and H_2O excretion, contracting the blood volume and reducing venous return to the heart.

INOTROPIC DRUGS

Digoxin is a glycoside extracted from foxglove leaves, *Digitalis* sp. It consists of a steroid ring structure (aglycone) which possesses the pharmacological activity, combined with sugar molecules (digitoxose) which enhance binding.

Mechanical effects and therapeutic benefit. Digoxin increases the force of cardiac contraction in the failing heart and reduces its oxygen consumption. This action is responsible for the therapeutic benefit of digitalis in heart failure. This benefit has often been doubted in patients with chronic heart failure in sinus rhythm, but recent clinical trials have shown that digoxin can reduce the symptoms of heart failure in patients who are already receiving diuretics. Digoxin is particularly indicated in heart failure due to atrial fibrillation (Chapter 17).

Mechanism of action. Digoxin inhibits membrane Na^+/K^+ ATPase (○), which is responsible for Na^+/K^+ exchange across the muscle cell membrane. This increases intracellular Na^+ and produces a secondary increase in intracellular Ca^{2+} which increases the force of myocardial contraction. The increase in intracellular Ca^{2+} occurs because the decreased Na^+ gradient across the membrane reduces the extrusion of Ca^{2+} by the Na^+/Ca^{2+} exchanger (○) that occurs during diastole.

Digoxin and K^+ ions compete for a 'receptor' (Na^+/K^+ ATPase) on the outside of the muscle cell membrane, so the effects of digoxin may be *dangerously increased in hypokalaemia*, produced, for example, by diuretics.

Electrical effects. These are due to a complicated mixture of direct and indirect actions.

Direct effects (bottom □). At non-toxic concentrations: (1) the cardiac action potential is shortened and the membrane resistance is lowered, probably because of the increased intracellular Ca^{2+}, which is known to increase the potassium conductance; (2) shortening of the action potential shortens the atrial and ventricular refractory period; and (3) toxic concentrations (top □) cause depolarization (due to Na^+ pump inhibition) and oscillatory depolarizing afterpotentials appear after normal action potentials (caused by increased intracellular Ca^{2+}). If the afterpotential reaches threshold, an action potential is generated causing an 'ectopic beat'. With increasing toxicity, the ectopic beat itself elicits further beats, causing a self-sustaining arrhythmia (ventricular tachycardia), which may progress to ventricular fibrillation.

Indirect effects. Digoxin increases central vagal activity and facilitates muscarinic transmission in the heart. This: (1) slows the heart rate; (2) slows atrioventricular conductance; and (3) prolongs the refractory period of the atrioventricular node and bundle of His. *Use is made of this effect in atrial fibrillation* (Chapter 17) but at toxic levels, heart block occurs.

Effects on other organs. Digoxin affects all excitable tissues, its cardioselectivity resulting from a greater dependence of myocardial function on the rate of sodium extrusion. The most common extracardiac action is on the gut and digoxin may cause anorexia, nausea, vomiting or diarrhoea. These effects are partly due to actions on the smooth muscle of the gut and partly a result of central vagal and chemoreceptor trigger zone stimulation. Less common effects include confusion or even psychosis.

Toxicity. Digoxin toxicity is *quite common.* According to its severity, treatment may require withdrawal of the drug, potassium supplements, antiarrhythmic drugs (phenytoin or lignocaine) or in very severe intoxication, digoxin-specific antibody fragments (Fab).

SYMPATHOMIMETIC AGENTS

These activate cardiac β_1-receptors and stimulate adenylyl cyclase, an effect mediated by a G-protein called G_s (left). The resulting rise in cAMP activates cAMP-dependent protein kinase which leads to phosphorylation of the L-type Ca^{2+} channels and an increase in the probability of their opening. This increases the influx of Ca^{2+} and hence the force of myocardial contraction. In general, they are little used in heart failure because they are arrhythmogenic and also increase the heart rate and oxygen consumption. This increases ischaemia and infarct size in myocardial infarction.

Dobutamine is given by intravenous infusion in *acute severe heart failure.* It stimulates β_1-adrenoceptors in the heart and increases contractility with little effect on rate.

Dopamine given by intravenous infusion also stimulates cardiac β_1-adrenoceptors. At lower doses, it increases renal perfusion by stimulating dopamine receptors in the renal vasculature. Dobutamine and low doses of dopamine are often given together in cardiogenic shock.

PHOSPHODIESTERASE INHIBITORS

Milrinone inhibits phosphodiesterase (PDE, left figure) in the myocardial cells causing a rise in intracellular cAMP and consequently an increase in Ca^{2+} influx. In addition to increasing myocardial contractility, milrinone is a vasodilator. It is given by intravenous infusion in severe congestive heart failure unresponsive to other therapy.

19 Drugs used to affect blood coagulation

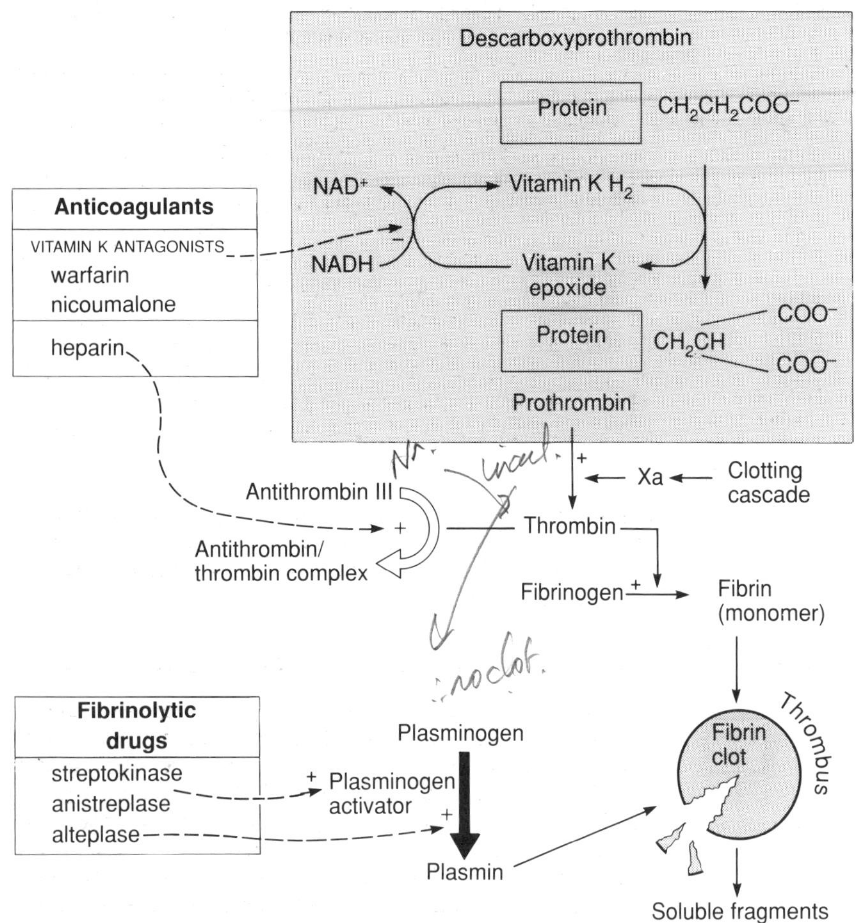

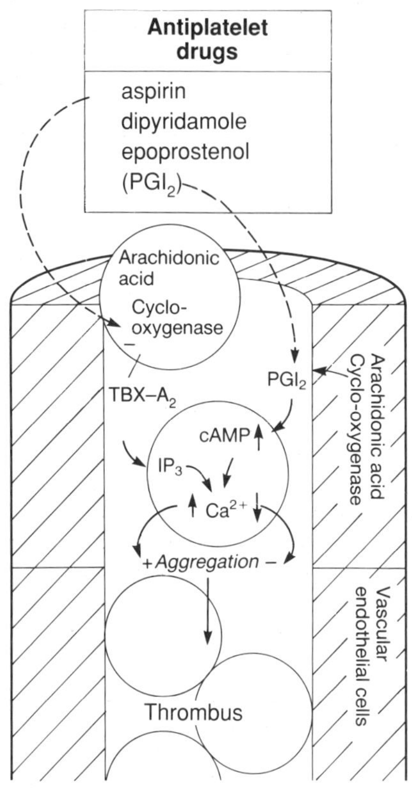

The centre of the figure shows the final stages of the cascade sequence involved in clot (thrombus) formation. In the slower-moving venous side of the circulation, the thrombus (○) consists of a fibrin web enmeshed with platelets and red blood cells. **Anticoagulant drugs** (top left), particularly heparin and warfarin, are widely used in the prevention and treatment of *venous thrombosis* and *embolism* (e.g. deep vein thrombosis, prevention of post-operative thrombosis, atrial fibrillation, patients with artifical heart valves). The main adverse effect of anticoagulants is **haemorrhage**.

Heparin is short-acting and must be given by injection. Its anticoagulant effect requires the presence of *antithrombin III*, a protease inhibitor in the blood that forms a 1:1 complex with thrombin (⇨). Heparin increases the *rate* of complex formation 1000-fold, causing the almost instantaneous inactivation of thrombin. In addition, the heparin–antithrombin III complex has inhibitory effects on factors IXa, Xa, XIa and XIIa. Heparin acts both *in vitro* and *in vivo*.

Warfarin is active orally. It is a coumarin derivative with a structure similar to that of vitamin K. Warfarin and some other anticoagulants (top left) block vitamin K-dependent γ-carboxylation of glutamate residues (top, shaded) resulting in the production of modified factors VII, IX, X and prothrombin. These are inactive in promoting coagulation because the γ-carboxylation confers Ca^{2+} binding properties which are essential for the proteins to assemble into an efficient catalytic complex. The oral anticoagulants are only active *in vivo* and take at least 36–48 hours for the anticoagulant effect to develop. Thus if an immediate effect is required, heparin must be given in addition.

Anticoagulants are less useful in preventing *arterial thrombosis*, because in faster-flowing vessels, thrombi are composed mainly of platelets with little fibrin. **Antiplatelet drugs** (right) may inhibit platelet aggregation and arterial thrombosis. **Aspirin** is the only drug for which there is convincing evidence of antiplatelet activity. It has been shown to be beneficial in ischaemic heart disease and especially in stroke prevention. Aspirin is thought to act by inhibiting the synthesis of platelet thromboxane-A_2 ($TBX-A_2$) (right figure) which is the major eicosanoid in platelets and a powerful inducer of aggregation.

Fibrinolytic drugs (bottom left) are administered intravenously. They are agents that can rapidly lyse thrombi by activating plasminogen to form plasmin (⬇), a proteolytic enzyme that degrades fibrin and so dissolves thrombi. Thrombolytic drugs, especially streptokinase are extensively used in the treatment of myocardial infarction and all have been shown to decrease mortality. The beneficial effects are greatest if the drugs are given within 3 hours of myocardial infarction, with progressively less benefit over 24 hours.

Thrombus is an unwanted clot inside a blood vessel. Thrombosis is particulary likely to occur where the blood flow is sluggish, because this allows activated clotting factors to accumulate instead of being washed away. A common problem is post-operative thrombosis in the leg veins. Sometimes bits of thrombus break off (emboli) and are carried to distant sites, which may be severly damaged e.g. pulmonary embolism. In atrial fibrillation, the loss of atrial contraction predisposes to stasis of blood and encourages thrombus formation. These may detach and cause cerebral embolism (stroke).

ANTICOAGULANTS

Heparin is a naturally occurring, highly acidic, glycosaminoglycan of varying molecular weight (5000–15 000). Subcutaneous injections or continuous intravenous infusions of heparin reduce the incidence of deep venous thrombosis in patients undergoing general surgery and those recovering from stroke and myocardial infarction.

The main side-effect of heparin is bleeding. This can usually be controlled by stopping the drug administration, since it has a short duration of action (4–6 hours). If necessary, heparin can be neutralized by the intravenous injection of protamine, a basic peptide that combines with the acidic heparin. Heparin occasionally causes allergic reactions and thrombocytopenia.

VITAMIN K ANTAGONISTS

Warfarin is well absorbed after oral administration, but the onset of its full anticoagulant effect is delayed for 1–3 days, while the inactive coagulation factors induced by the drug gradually replace those originally present. Warfarin has a long half-life (about 40 hours) and it can take up to 5 days for the prothrombin time to return to normal after stopping treatment. It is metabolized by the liver to inactive 7-hydroxywarfarin. Drugs that induce hepatic microsomal enzymes (e.g. *barbiturates*, *carbamazepine*) antagonize the anticoagulant action of warfarin, and haemorrhage may occur if they are withdrawn. Drugs that inhibit hepatic enzymes decrease the catabolism of warfarin and potentiate its action (e.g. *cimetidine*, *ethanol*, *metronidazole*). Warfarin can be reversed by giving a concentrate of clotting factors (or fresh frozen plasma which contains clotting factors) and is the treatment of choice for rapid reversal. In severe overdosage, vitamin K (phytomenadione) can be given by intravenous injection but takes 6–12 hours to act.

ANTIPLATELET DRUGS

Aspirin is widely used in the prophylaxis of myocardial infarction and stroke. Clinical trials have shown that aspirin reduces the probability of experiencing a second myocardial infarction. There is also some evidence that an alternate day dose of aspirin can reduce the incidence of primary myocardial infarction. The beneficial effects of aspirin in thromboembolic disease are thought to be due to the inhibition of platelet thromboxane-A_2 (TBX-A_2) synthesis. Thromboxane-A_2 is a powerful inducer of platelet aggregation. It acts on cell surface receptors and activates phospholipase C, causing the formation of second messengers (inositol triphosphate, IP_3 and diacylglycerol, DG; Chapter 1) and consequently a rise in intracellular calcium which triggers aggregation. The endothelial cells of the vascular wall produce a prostaglandin, PGI_2 (prostacyclin) which may be the physiological antagonist of TBX-A_2. PGI_2 stimulates different receptors on the platelet and activates adenylyl cyclase. The resulting increase in cAMP is associated with a decrease in intracellular calcium and inhibition of platelet aggregation. Aspirin prevents TBX-A_2 formation by irreversibly inhibiting cyclo-oxygenase (Chapter 30). Platelets cannot synthesize new enzyme, but the vascular endothelial cells can, and aspirin (320 mg day^{-1}) given on alternate days produces a selective inhibition of cyclo-oxygenase over much of the dose interval. Thus, the balance of the anti-aggregatory effects of PGI_2 and the pro-aggregatory effects of TBX-A_2 is shifted in a beneficial direction.

Dipyridamole is used with warfarin to prevent thrombosis formation on prosthetic heart valves. The mechanism of action of dipyridamole is unknown and it is of doubtful efficacy. (It has no effect on its own.)

FIBRINOLYTIC DRUGS (THROMBOLYTICS)

Fibrinolytic drugs (mainly streptokinase) are used extensively in myocardial infarction to lyse the thrombi that block coronary arteries. They are administered by intravenous infusion and probably cause reperfusion in about 50% of arteries, if given within 3 hours. *The beneficial effects of aspirin in myocardial infarction are additive to those of streptokinase.* The main side-effects of thrombolytics are nausea, vomiting, bleeding and, except for alteplase, allergic reactions. Bleeding is usually restricted to the injection site but occasionally stroke occurs. **Streptokinase** is not an enzyme, it binds to circulating plasminogen to form an activator complex which converts further plasminogen to plasmin. Because there is a large excess of plasmin inhibitors in the blood, which can neutralize circulating plasmin, bleeding is not usually a problem. Within the thrombus, the concentration of plasmin inhibitors is low, and so streptokinase has some selectivity for clots. However, the increased circulating plasmin also digests fibrinogen and prothrombin, and the drug therefore has an additional anticoagulant effect.

Alteplase is natural plasminogen activator produced by recombinant DNA technology. Alteplase does not cause allergic reactions and can be used in patients when recent streptococcal infections or recent use of streptokinase contraindicates the use of streptokinase (i.e. patients at some risk of anaphylaxis).

Anistreplase (anisoylated plasminogen–streptokinase activator complex: APSAC) is a complex of human plasminogen and streptokinase made inactive by an anisoyl group at the catalytic centre. In the blood, the anisoyl group is slowly lost to give active plasminogen–streptokinase. This lengthens the duration of action to 4–6 hours and allows it to be given as a single intravenous injection. Because it contains streptokinase, allergic reactions may occur.

20 Agents used in anaemias

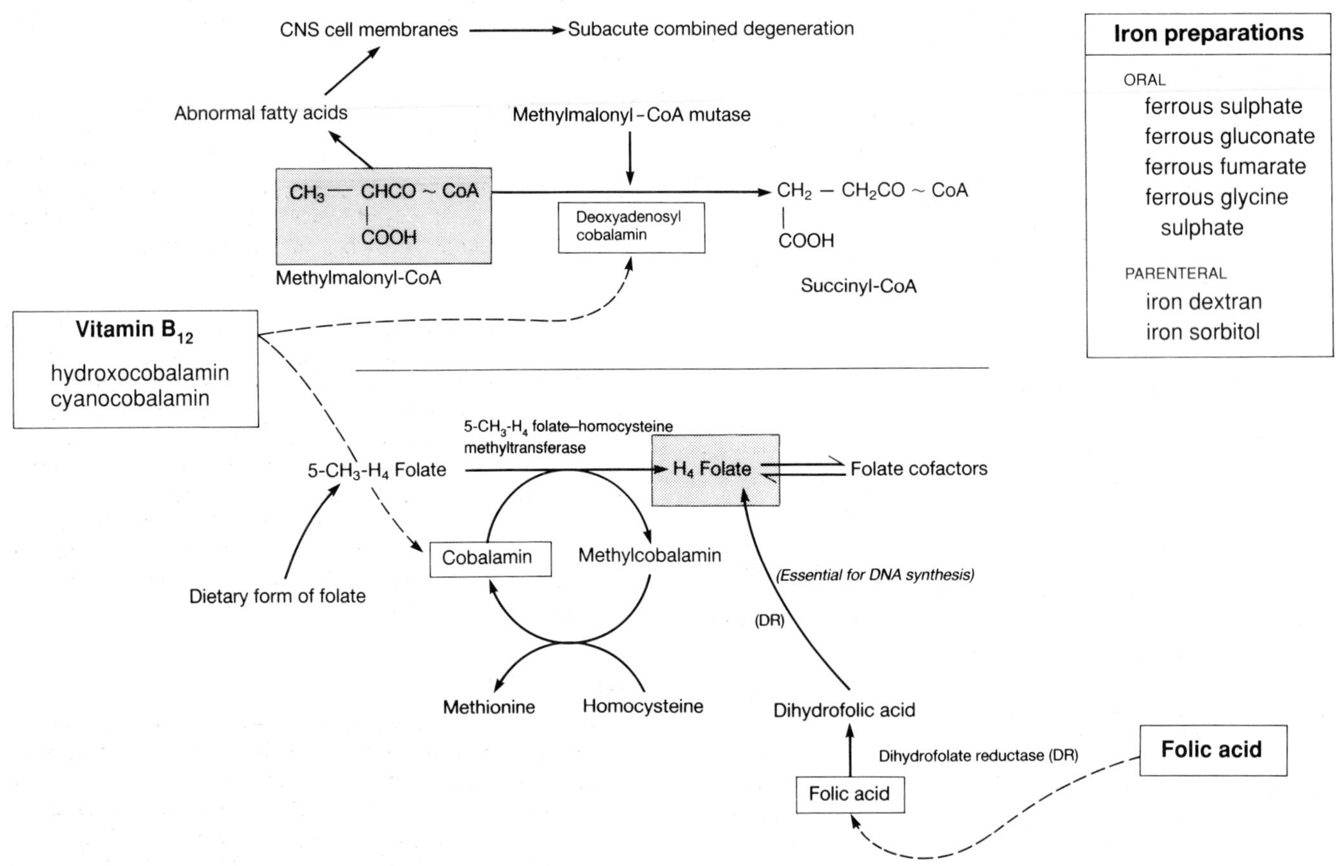

Normal erythropoiesis requires iron, vitamin B_{12} and folic acid. A deficiency of any of these causes anaemia. Erythropoietic activity is regulated by **erythropoietin**, a hormone released mainly by the kidneys. In chronic renal failure, anaemia often occurs due to a fall in erythropoietin production.

Iron is necessary for haemoglobin production and iron deficiency results in small red blood cells with insufficient haemoglobin (microcytic hypochromic anaemia). The administration of iron preparations (top right) is needed in iron deficiency, which may be due to chronic blood loss, pregnancy (the fetus takes iron from the mother), various abnormalities of the gut (iron absorption may be reduced) or premature birth (such babies are born with very low iron stores).

The main problem with oral iron preparations is that they frequently cause *gastrointestinal upsets*. Oral therapy is continued until haemoglobin is normal and the body stores of iron are built up by several months of lower iron doses. Children are very sensitive to iron toxicity and can be killed by the ingestion of as few as 10 tablets.

Vitamin B_{12} and **folic acid** are essential for several reactions necessary for normal DNA synthesis. A deficiency of either vitamin causes impaired production and abnormal maturation of erythroid precursor cells (megaloblastic anaemia). In addition to anaemia, vitamin B_{12} deficiency causes *central nervous system degeneration* (subacute combined degeneration), which may result in psychiatric or physical symptoms. The anaemia is due to a block of H_4 folate synthesis (lower figure, ▢) and the nervous degeneration is due to an accumulation of methylmalonyl-CoA (upper figure, ▢).

Vitamin B_{12} deficiency occurs when there is malabsorption due to lack of intrinsic factor (pernicious anaemia), following gastrectomy (no intrinsic factor), or in various small-bowel diseases, where absorption is impaired. Since the disease is nearly always due to malabsorption, oral vitamin administration is of little value, and replacement therapy, usually for life, involves injections of vitamin B_{12} (left). Hydroxocobalamin is the form of choice for therapy because it is retained in the body longer than cyanocobalamin (cyanocobalamin is bound less to plasma proteins and is more rapidly excreted in the urine).

Folic acid deficiency leading to a megaloblastic anaemia, which requires oral folic acid (bottom right), may occur in pregnancy (folate requirement is increased) and in malabsorption syndromes (e.g. steatorrhoea and sprue).

IRON

The nucleus of haem is formed by iron, which, in combination with the appropriate globin chains, forms the protein haemoglobin. Over 90% of the non-storage iron in the body is in haemoglobin (about 2.3 g). Some iron (about 1 g) is stored as ferritin and haemosiderin in macrophages in the spleen, liver and bone marrow.

Absorption. Iron is normally absorbed in the duodenum and proximal jejunum. Normally 5–10% of dietary iron is absorbed (about 0.5–1 mg day^{-1}) but this can be increased if iron stores are low. Iron must be in the ferrous form for absorption, which occurs by active transport. In the plasma, iron is transported bound to transferrin, a β-globulin. There is no mechanism for excretion of iron and regulation of iron balance is achieved by appropriate changes in iron absorption.

IRON PREPARATIONS

For oral therapy, iron preparations contain ferrous salts, because these are absorbed most efficiently. In iron-deficient patients, about 50–100 mg of iron can be incorporated into haemoglobin daily. Since about 25% of oral ferrous salts can be absorbed, 200–400 mg iron should be given daily for the fastest possible correction of deficiency. If this causes intolerable gastrointestinal irritation (nausea, epigastric pain, diarrhoea, constipation), lower doses can be given, which will completely correct the iron deficiency, but more slowly.

Parenteral iron should only be used if oral therapy has failed. It does not hasten the haemoglobin response.

Iron dextran is a complex of iron hydroxide with high molecular weight dextrans. It is usually given in a series of deep intramuscular injections, but can be given in one dose by intravenous infusion. Side-effects include vomiting, transient nausea and, rarely, severe anaphylaxis.

Iron sorbitol is a complex of iron, sorbitol and citric acid. It is not suitable for intravenous injection.

Iron toxicity. Acute toxicity occurs most commonly in young children who have ingested iron tablets. These cause necrotizing gastroenteritis, with abdominal pain, vomiting, bloody diarrhoea and, later, shock. This may be followed, even after apparent improvement, by acidosis, coma and death.

VITAMIN B_{12}

In megaloblastic anaemias, the underlying defect is impaired DNA synthesis. Cell division is decreased, but RNA and protein synthesis continue. This results in large (macrocytic) fragile red cells. The cobalt atom at the centre of the vitamin B_{12} molecule covalently binds different ligands, forming various cobalamins. *Methylcobalamin* and *deoxyadenosylcobalamin* are the active forms of the vitamin and other cobalamins must be converted to these active forms.

Vitamin B_{12} (extrinsic factor) is absorbed only when complexed with *intrinsic factor*, a glycoprotein secreted by the *parietal cells* of the gastric mucosa. Absorption occurs in the distal ileum by a highly specific transport process and the vitamin is then transported bound to transcobalamin II (a plasma glycoprotein). *Pernicious anaemia* results from a *deficiency* in intrinsic factor caused by autoantibodies, either to the factor itself or to the gastric parietal cells (atrophic gastritis).

Methylmalonyl-CoA mutase. This enzyme requires deoxyadenosylcobalamin for the conversion of methylmalonyl-CoA to succinyl-CoA. In the absence of vitamin B_{12}, this reaction cannot take place and there is accumulation of *methylmalonyl-CoA*. This results in the synthesis of abnormal fatty acids, which become incorporated in neuronal membranes and cause the neurological defects seen in vitamin B_{12} deficiency.

5-CH_3-H_4 folate-homocysteine methyltransferase converts 5-CH_3-H_4 folate and homocysteine to H_4 folate and methionine. In this reaction, cobalamin is converted to methylcobalamin. When vitamin B_{12} deficiency prevents this reaction, the conversion of the major dietary and storage folate (5-CH_3-H_4 folate) to the precursor of folate cofactors (H_4 folate) cannot occur and a deficiency in the folate cofactors necessary for DNA synthesis develops. This reaction links folic acid and vitamin B_{12} metabolism and explains why high doses of folic acid can improve the anaemia, but not the nervous degeneration, caused by vitamin B_{12} deficiency.

FOLIC ACID

The body stores of folates are relatively low (5–20 mg) and as daily requirements are high, folic acid deficiency and megaloblastic anaemia can quickly develop (1–6 months) if the intake of folic acid stops. Folic acid itself is completely absorbed in the proximal jejunum, but dietary folates are mainly polyglutamate forms of 5-CH_3-H_4 folate. All but one of the glutamyl residues are hydrolysed off before the absorption of monoglutamate 5-CH_3-H_4 folate. In contrast to vitamin B_{12} deficiency, folic acid deficiency is often caused by inadequate dietary intake of folate. Some drugs (e.g. *phenytoin, oral contraceptives, isoniazid*) can cause folic acid deficiency by reducing its absorption.

Folic acid and vitamin B_{12} have no known toxic effects. However, it is important not to give folic acid alone in vitamin B_{12} deficiency states, because although the anaemia may improve, the neurological degeneration progresses and may become irreversible.

ERYTHROPOIETIN

Hypoxia, or loss of blood, results in increased haemoglobin synthesis and release of erythrocytes. These changes are mediated by an increase in circulating erythropoietin (a glycoprotein containing 166 amino acid residues). Recombinant erythropoietin (r-HuEPO) has recently become available and has been shown to be very effective (when given by intravenous or subcutaneous injection) in correcting the anaemia of renal disease, which is caused largely by a deficiency of the hormone.

21 Central transmitter substances

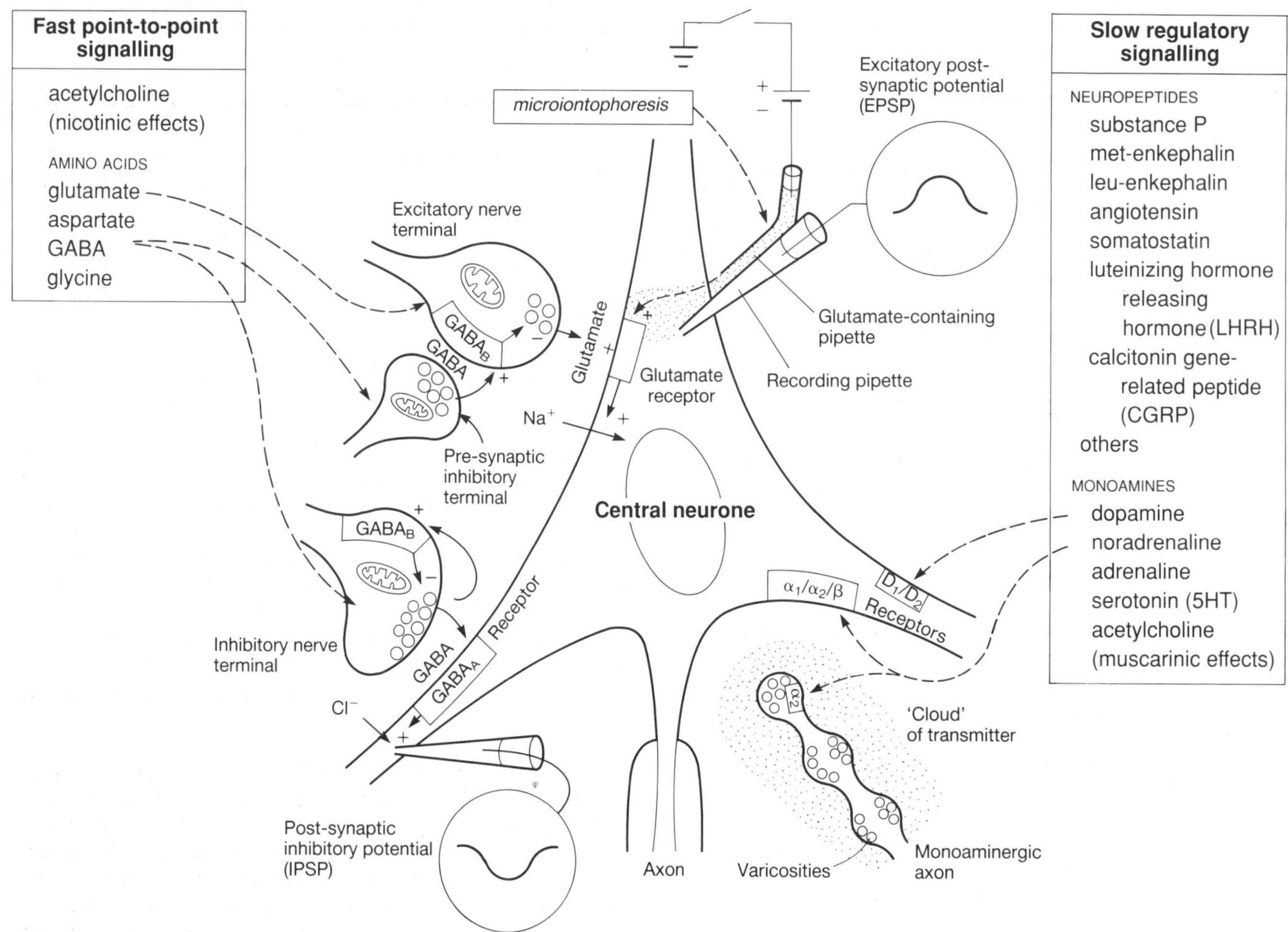

Drugs acting on the central nervous system are used more than any other type of agent. In addition to their therapeutic uses, drugs such as *caffeine*, *alcohol* and *nicotine* are used socially to provide a sense of well-being. Central drugs often produce dependence with continued use (Chapter 29) and many are subject to strict legal controls.

The mechanisms by which central drugs produce their therapeutic effects are usually unknown, reflecting our lack of understanding of neurological and psychiatric disease. Knowledge of central transmitter substances is important because virtually all drugs acting on the brain produce their effects by modifying synaptic transmission.

The transmitters used in fast, point-to-point neural circuits are **amino acids** (left) except for a few cholinergic synapses with nicotinic receptors. *Glutamate* is the main central excitatory transmitter. It depolarizes neurones by triggering an increase in membrane Na^+ conductance. *γ-Aminobutyric acid* (GABA) is the main inhibitory transmitter, perhaps being released at one-third of all central synapses. It hyperpolarizes neurones by increasing their membrane Cl^- conductance and stabilizes the resting membrane potential near the Cl^- equilibrium potential. *Glycine* is also an inhibitory transmitter, mainly in the spinal cord.

In addition to fast point-to-point signalling, the brain possesses more diffuse regulatory systems, which use **monoamines** as their transmitters (bottom right). The cell bodies of these branched axons project to many areas of the brain. Transmitter release occurs diffusely from many points along varicose terminal networks of monoaminergic neurones, affecting very large numbers of target cells. The functions of the central monoaminergic pathways are obscure, but they are involved in disorders such as *Parkinsonism*, *depression*, *migraine* and *schizophrenia*.

Most recently, many **peptides** (top right) have been found in central neurones and nerve terminals. The evidence for their role as transmitter substances is usually very incomplete. They probably form another group of diffusely acting regulatory transmitters, but as yet the physiological roles of most of them are unknown.

Microiontophoresis is a method of applying drugs locally to neurones by the passage of electrical current. By combining drug-containing micropipettes with a recording electrode, the effects of agonists and antagonists on neurones can be studied and compared with endogenous transmitter, released by appropriate nerve stimulation. This technique has been used extensively in the study of central transmitters and drugs.

AMINO ACIDS

GABA is present in all areas of the central nervous system, mainly in local inhibitory interneurones. It rapidly inhibits central neurones, the response being mediated by post-synaptic $GABA_A$ receptors, which are blocked by the convulsant drug bicuculline. Some GABA receptors ($GABA_B$) are not blocked by bicuculline, but are selectively activated by baclofen (*p*-chlorophenyl-GABA). Although $GABA_B$-receptor antagonists exist (e.g. phaclofen), their lack of potency has made it difficult to establish the physiological role of $GABA_B$ receptors. Nevertheless, it is clear that many $GABA_B$ receptors are located on presynaptic nerve terminals and their activation results in a reduction in transmitter release (e.g. of glutamate and GABA itself). Baclofen reduces glutamate release in the spinal cord and produces an antispastic effect, which is useful in controlling the muscular spasms that occur in diseases such as multiple sclerosis.

Following release from presynaptic nerve terminals, amino acid transmitters are inactivated by reuptake systems.

Drugs which are thought to act by modifying GABAergic synaptic transmission include the *benzodiazepines*, *barbiturates* (Chapter 23) and the anticonvulsants *vigabatrin* and perhaps *valproate* (Chapter 24).

Glycine is an inhibitory transmitter in spinal interneurones. It is antagonized by strychnine and its release is prevented by tetanus toxin, both substances causing convulsions.

Glutamate (and **aspartate**) excite virtually all central neurones by activating several types of excitatory amino acid receptor. These receptors are classified into kainate, AMPA* and NMDA* receptors depending whether or not they are selectively activated by these glutamate analogues. No therapeutic drug is known to produce its effects by acting specifically at glutamate synapses. However, NMDA receptor antagonists (e.g. 2-aminophosphonovalerate) have been shown to have anticonvulsant activity in many experimental animal models of epilepsy and they may prove to be beneficial in stroke, where at least some of the neuronal damage is thought to result from an excessive release of glutamate.

MONOAMINES

Acetylcholine is mainly excitatory in the brain. It is the transmitter released from motoneurone nerve endings at the neuromuscular junction and at collateral axon synapses with Renshaw cells in the spinal cord. This provides the best example of a central nicotinic synapse. The excitatory effects of acetylcholine on central neurones are usually mediated via muscarinic receptors and may involve suppression of a voltage-sensitive K^+ conductance (M current). This inhibition increases the excitability of the cell and facilitates its response to tonic excitatory influences.

Cholinergic neurones are particularly abundant in the basal ganglia and others seem to be involved in cortical arousal responses and in memory. *Atropine-like* drugs can impair memory and the amnesic action of hyoscine is made use of in anaesthetic premedication (Chapter 22). They are also used for their central actions in *motion sickness* and *Parkinsonism* (Chapter 25). Loss of cholinergic neurones and memory are prominant features of *Alzheimer's disease*, a common form of senile dementia for which there is no effective treatment at present.

Catecholamines generally have inhibitory effects when applied locally onto central neurones.

Dopamine pathways project from the *substantia nigra* in the midbrain to the basal ganglia and from the *midbrain* to the limbic cortex and other limbic structures. A third (tuberoinfundibular) pathway is involved in regulating prolactin release. The nigrostriatal pathway is concerned with modulating the control of voluntary movement and its degeneration results in *Parkinsonism*. The mesolimbic pathway is 'overactive' in *schizophrenia*, but it is not known why. Dopamine *agonists* are used in the treatment of Parkinsonism (Chapter 25) and *antagonists* (neuroleptics) are used in schizophrenia (Chapter 26).

Noradrenaline-containing cell bodies occur in several groups in the brainstem. The largest of these nuclei is the *locus coeruleus* in the pons which projects to the entire dorsal forebrain, especially the cerebral cortex and hippocampus. The hypothalamus also possesses a high density of noradrenergic fibres. Noradrenaline and dopamine in limbic forebrain structures (especially the nucleus accumbens) may be involved in an ascending 'reward' system which has been implicated in *drug dependence* (Chapter 29). Impairment of noradrenergic function may be associated with *depression* (Chapter 27).

Serotonin (5-hydroxytryptamine, 5HT) occurs in cell bodies in the *raphe nucleus* of the brainstem which projects to many forebrain areas and to the ventral and dorsal horns of the spinal cord. The latter, descending, projection may modulate pain inputs (Chapter 28). Serotonin has been implicated in the sleep–wake cycle, temperature control and the control of aggressive behaviour. Serotonin may, like noradrenaline, be involved in *depression*.

Adrenaline is of minor importance in the brain, but innervation of the nucleus tractus solitarius may play an important role in central *blood pressure control* (Chapter 15).

Neuropeptides form the most numerous group of possible central transmitters, but little is known yet of their functions. Substance P and the enkephalins are thought to be involved in pain pathways (Chapter 28).

* AMPA, α-amino-3-hydroxy-5-methyl-4-isoxazolepropionic acid; NMDA, *N*-methyl-D-aspartate.

22 General anaesthetics

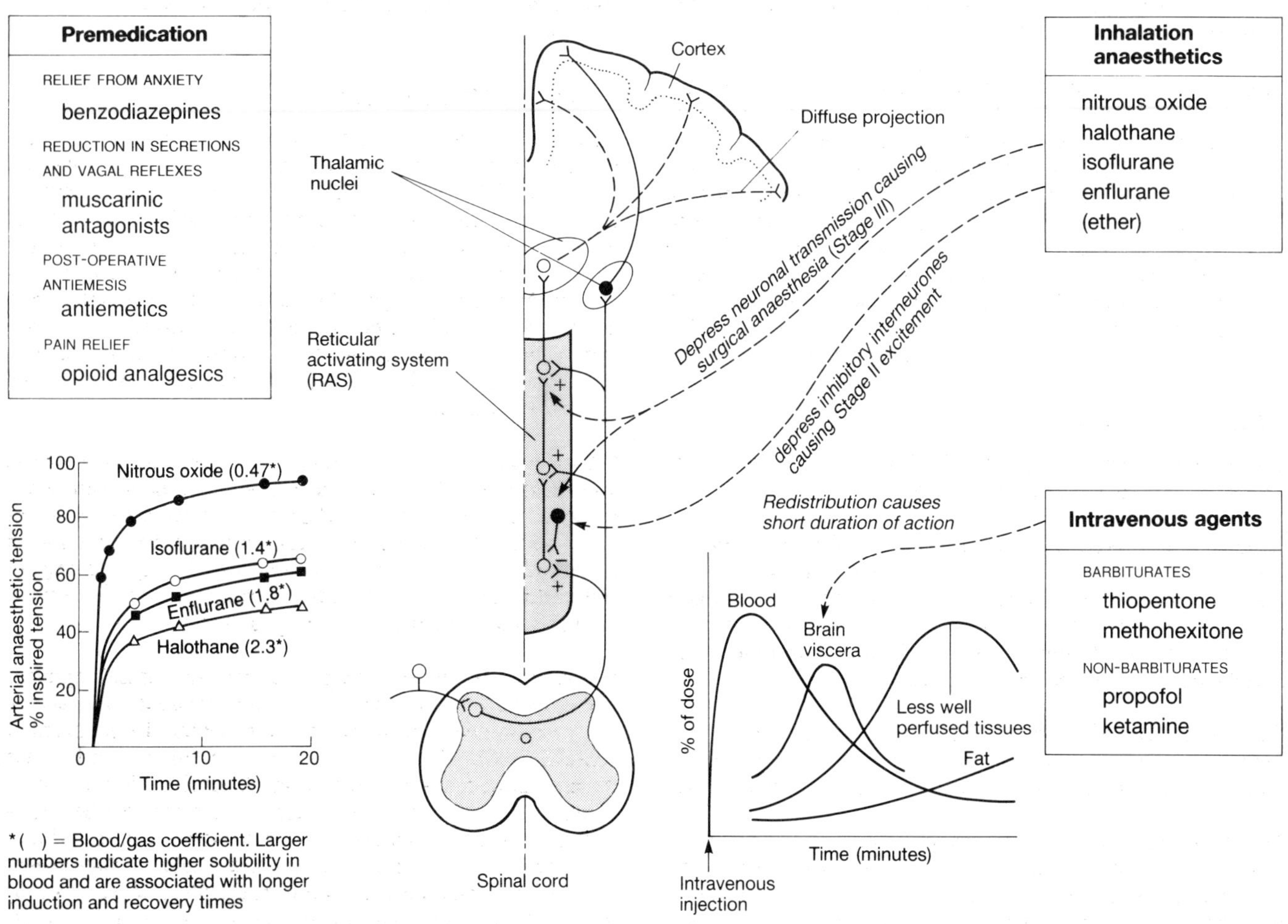

General anaesthesia is the absence of sensation associated with a reversible loss of consciousness. Numerous agents ranging from inert gases to steroids produce anaesthesa in animals, but only a few are used clinically (right). Historical anaesthetics include ether, chloroform, cyclopropane, ethylchloride and trichlorethylene.

Anaesthetics depress all excitable tissues including central neurones, cardiac muscle and smooth and striatal muscle. However, these tissues have different sensitivities to anaesthetics and the areas of the brain responsible for consciousness (middle, ☐) are among the most sensitive. Thus, it is possible to administer anaesthetic agents at concentrations that produce unconsciousness without unduly depressing the cardiovascular and respiratory centres or the myocardium. However, for most anaesthetics, *the margin of safety is small.*

General anaesthesia usually involves the administration of different drugs for **premedication** (top left), **induction** of anaesthesia (bottom right) and **maintenance** of anaesthesia (top right). Premedication has two main aims: (1) the prevention of the parasympathomimetic effects of anaesthesia (bradycardia, bronchial secretion); and (2) the reduction of anxiety or pain.

Induction is most commonly achieved by the intravenous injection of **thiopentone** or **propofol**. Unconsciousness occurs within seconds and is maintained by the administration of an inhalation anaesthetic. **Halothane** is a widely used volatile anaesthetic in the UK, but it is associated with a very low incidence of post-operative hepatitis. **Enflurane** and **isoflurane** are newer agents that are being used increasingly because they are not hepatotoxic. **Nitrous oxide** at concentrations up to 70% in oxygen is the most widely used anaesthetic agent. It is used with oxygen as a carrier gas, for the volatile agents, or together with opioid analgesics (e.g. *fentanyl*). Nitrous oxide causes sedation and analgesia but it is not sufficient alone to maintain anaesthesia.

During the induction of anaesthesia, distinct 'stages' occur with some agents, especially ether. First, analgesia is produced (Stage I), followed by excitement (Stage II) caused by inhibition of inhibitory reticular neurones (•—<). Then surgical anaesthesia (Stage III) develops, the depth of which depends on the amount of drug administered. These stages are not obvious with currently used anaesthetics.

Reticular activating system (RAS). This is a complex polysynaptic pathway in the brainstem reticular formation that projects diffusely to the cortex. Activity in the RAS is concerned with maintaining consciousness and because it is especially sensitive to the depressant action of anaesthetics, it is thought to be their primary site of action.

Mechanism of action of anaesthetics. It is not known how anaesthetics produce their effects. Anaesthetic potency correlates well with lipid solubility and anaesthetics may dissolve in the lipid bilayer of the cell membrane, expanding the membrane and increasing its fluidity. The resulting disorder in the membrane may alter ionic fluxes (decrease sodium influx or increase potassium efflux) and produce anaesthesia. A finding consistant with this idea is that high pressure reverses anaesthesia, presumably by 'reordering' the cell membrane. A minority view is that anaesthetics might bind to a hydrophobic area of a protein and inhibit its normal function.

PREMEDICATION

Relief from anxiety (Chapter 23). Oral *benzodiazepines* such as diazepam or lorazepam are most effective.

Reduction in secretions and vagal reflexes. *Muscarinic antagonists*, usually atropine or hyoscine, are used to prevent salivation and bronchial secretions, and more importantly to protect the heart from arrhythmias, particularly bradycardia caused by halothane, suxamethonium and neostigmine. Hyoscine is also antiemetic and produces some amnesia.

Analgesics. *Opioid analgesics* (Chapter 28) are often given before an operation, particularly morphine. Fentanyl and related drugs are used to supplement nitrous oxide anaesthesia.

Post-operative antiemesis. Nausea and vomiting are very common after anaesthesia. Often opioid drugs given during and after the operation are responsible. Sometimes antiemetic drugs (e.g. droperidol, metoclopramide, prochlorperazine) are given with the premedication, but they are more effective if administered intravenously during anaesthesia.

INTRAVENOUS AGENTS

These may be used alone for short surgical procedures, but are used mainly for the induction of anaesthesia.

Barbiturates. *Thiopentone* injected intravenously induces anaesthesia in less than 30 seconds because the very lipid-soluble drug quickly dissolves in the rapidly perfused brain. Recovery from thiopentone is rapid because of redistribution into less-perfused tissues (bottom right figure). Thiopentone is subsequently metabolized by the liver at a rate of 12–16% per hour. Doses of thiopentone only slightly above the 'sleep dose' depress the myocardium and the respiratory centre. Very occasionally anaphylaxis may occur. *Methohexitone* has similar actions to thiopentone, but is shorter acting and may produce pain on injection.

Non-barbiturates. Many agents with potential advantages over the barbiturates (e.g. less myocardial depression, more rapid elimination) have been introduced, but few have found much favour for long. *Propofol* (2,6-diisopropylphenol) is associated with rapid recovery without nausea or hangover and for this reason is increasingly used. It may, however, occasionally cause convulsions and, very rarely, anaphylaxis. *Ketamine* may cause nightmares.

INHALATION AGENTS

Uptake and distribution (bottom left figure). The speed at which induction of anaesthesia occurs depends mainly on its *solubility in blood* and the *inspired concentration* of gas. When agents of low solubility (nitrous oxide) diffuse from the lungs into arterial blood, relatively small amounts are required to saturate the blood, and so the arterial tension (and hence brain tension) rises quickly. More soluble agents (halothane) require the solution of much more anaesthetic before the arterial anaesthetic tension approaches that of the inspired gas and so induction is slower. Recovery from anaesthesia is also slower with increasing anaesthetic solubility.

Nitrous oxide is not potent enough to use as a sole anaesthetic agent, but it is commonly used as a non-flammable carrier gas for volatile agents, allowing their concentration to be significantly reduced. It is a good analgesic and a 50% mixture in oxygen (Entonox) is used when analgesia is required (e.g. in childbirth, road traffic accidents). Nitrous oxide has little effect on the cardiovascular or respiratory systems.

Halothane ($CF_3CHBrCl$) is a potent agent and, as the vapour is non-irritant, induction is smooth and pleasant. It causes a concentration-dependent hypotension, largely by myocardial depression. Halothane often causes arrhythmias and because the myocardium is sensitized to catecholamines, infiltration of adrenaline may cause cardiac arrest. Like most volatile anaesthetics, halothane depresses the respiratory centre, with a resulting decrease in the minute volume and an increase in arterial P_{CO_2}. The most important toxic effect of halothane is massive hepatic necrosis which occurs in about 1 in 35 000 cases, although lesser degrees of liver damage probably occur much more often. More than 20% of the administered halothane is biotransformed by the liver to metabolites, some of which may either directly damage the liver or bind to cellular macromolecules and generate antigens that are recognized as foreign by the body.

Enflurane ($F_2HC\text{-}O\text{-}CF_2\text{-}CHFCl$) is similar in action to halothane. It also depresses myocardial contractility and causes a dose-dependent hypotension. However, there is a much lower incidence of arrhythmias than with halothane and much less sensitization of the myocardium to catecholamines. Enflurane undergoes much less metabolism (2%) than halothane and is unlikely to cause hepatitis. The disadvantage of enflurane is that it may cause seizure activity in the EEG and, occasionally, muscle twitching.

Isoflurane ($F_3CCHCl\text{-}O\text{-}CF_2H$) has similar actions to halothane but is less cardiodepressant and does not sensitize the heart to adrenaline. It causes dose-related hypotension by decreasing systemic vascular resistance. Only 0.2% of the absorbed dose is metabolized and so isoflurane is very unlikely to cause hepatitis.

23 Anxiolytics and hypnotics

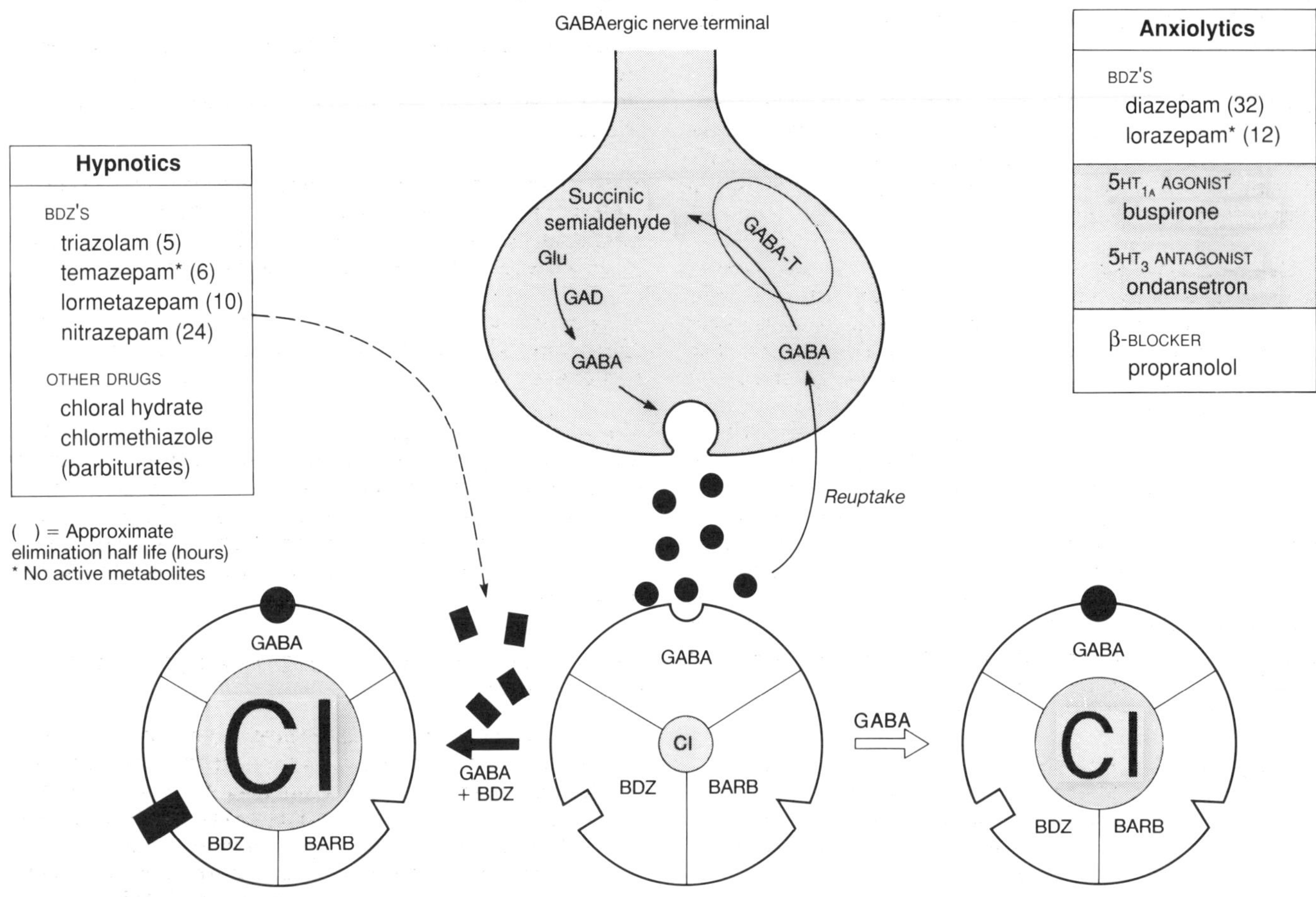

Drug treatment of *sleep disorders* (hypnotics) and *anxiety states* (anxiolytics) is dominated by the **benzodiazepines** (BDZs). In general, these drugs will induce sleep when given in high doses at night and will provide sedation and reduce anxiety when given in low, divided doses during the day.

Benzodiazepines have *anxiolytic*, *hypnotic*, *muscle relaxant* and *anticonvulsant* actions which are thought to be caused, at least in part, by the enhancement of *GABA-mediated inhibition* in the central nervous system. GABA (●) released from nerve terminals (top middle, shaded) binds to **$GABA_A$ receptors** (bottom middle) the activation of which increases the Cl^- conductance of the neurone (bottom right). The $GABA_A/Cl^-$ channel complex also has BDZ and barbiturate (BARB) modulatory receptor sites (bottom). Occupation of the BDZ sites by benzodiazepine receptor agonists (▬) enhances the actions of GABA on the Cl^- conductance of the neuronal membrane (bottom left). The **barbiturates** similarly enhance the action of GABA (not illustrated).

The popularity of benzodiazepines arose from their apparently low toxicity, but it is now realized that chronic benzodiazepine treatment may cause cognitive impairment, tolerance and **dependence**. Thus, the use of benzodiazepines in anxiety is decreasing, and the importance of using them only for the short-term relief (2–4 weeks) of severe anxiety or insomnia is being emphasized. Some new drugs which act on central **serotonergic receptors** (right, ☐) lack the adverse effects of benzodiazepines and may prove to be useful anxiolytics.

Different benzodiazepines are marketed as hypnotics (top left) and anxiolytics (top right). It is mainly the duration of action that determines the choice of drug. Many benzodiazepines are metabolized in the liver to **active metabolites**, which may have longer elimination half-lives ($t_{\frac{1}{2}}$) than the parent drug. For example, diazepam ($t_{\frac{1}{2}} \simeq$ 20–80 hours) has an active *N*-desmethyl metabolite which has an elimination half-life of up to 200 hours.

Benzodiazepines used as hypnotics can be divided into two groups: (1) short acting (top left); and (2) longer acting (middle left). A rapidly eliminated drug (e.g. temazepam) is usually preferred to avoid daytime sedation. A longer-acting drug (e.g. nitrazepam) might be preferred where early morning waking is a problem and where a daytime anxiolytic effect is needed.

GABAergic nerve terminals. Around 30–50% of synapses on the brain are believed to be GABAergic. The vast majority of GABAergic neurones are short interneurones.

GAD (L-glutamic acid decarboxylase) catalyses the synthesis of GABA from glutamate. It is concentrated in the GABAergic nerve terminals.

GABA-T (GABA-ketoglutarate transaminase) inactivates GABA by transamination to succinate semialdehyde (SSA), which is then oxidized to succinate. Inhibitors of GABA-T increase brain GABA levels and one, γ-vinyl-GABA is used in refractory epilepsy (Chapter 24).

GABA receptors (Chapter 21) of the $GABA_A$ type are involved in the actions of hypnotics/anxiolytics. The $GABA_A$ receptor belongs to the superfamily of ligand-gated ion channels (other examples are the nicotinic, glycine and $5HT_3$ receptors). The $GABA_A$ receptor consists of several subunits (α, β, γ and δ) and variants of each of these subunits have been cloned (six α-, three β- and two γ-subunits, had been sequenced by the end of 1991). The subunit compositions of natural $GABA_A$ receptors in the brain are unknown. If the $GABA_A$ receptor is pentameric, (like the nicotinic receptor) then a major type is probably $2\alpha_1\ 2\beta_2, \gamma_2$ because mRNAs encoding these subunits are often colocalized in the brain. Electrophysiological experiments on toad oocytes possessing various combinations of $GABA_A$ subunits (produced by injecting their mRNA into the oocyte) have revealed that receptors constructed from α- and β-subunits respond to GABA (*g*Cl increases), but for a receptor to respond to a benzodiazepine a γ-subunit is required.

Recently, compounds have been discovered that are *antagonists* or *partial agonists* at the benzodiazepine receptors. Others actually increase anxiety and are called *inverse agonists*. It remains to be seen whether the development of partial agonists will lead to a non-sedative anxiolytic.

Flumazenil is a competitive benzodiazepine antagonist that has a short duration of action and is given intravenously. It can be used to reverse the sedative effects of benzodiazepines in anaesthetic, intensive care and diagnostic procedures.

Barbiturate receptor. Barbiturates increase GABA-mediated inhibition by prolonging the duration of individual Cl^- channel openings triggered by a given GABA stimulus (benzodiazepines increase the frequency of Cl^- channel opening). Barbiturates are far more depressant than benzodiazepines because at higher doses they may increase the Cl^- conductance directly and decrease the sensitivity of the neuronal post-synaptic membrane to excitatory transmitters.

Barbiturates were extensively used, but are now obsolete as hypnotics and anxiolytics because they readily lead to psychological and physical dependence, induce microsomal enzymes, and relatively small overdosage may be fatal. In contrast, huge overdoses of benzodiazepines have been taken without serious long-term effects. Barbiturates (e.g. thiopentone, Chapter 22) remain important in anaesthesia and are still used as anticonvulsants (e.g. phenobarbitone, Chapter 24).

BENZODIAZEPINES (BDZs)

These are active orally and although most are metabolized by oxidation in the liver, they do not induce hepatic enzyme systems. They are central depressants, but in contrast to other hypnotics and anxiolytics, their maximum effect when given orally does not normally cause fatal, or even severe, respiratory depression. However, respiratory depression may occur in patients with bronchopulmonary disease or with intravenous administration.

Adverse effects include drowsiness, impaired alertness, agitation and ataxia, especially in the elderly. Triazolam may produce additional psychiatric disturbances and is best avoided.

Dependence. A physical withdrawal syndrome may occur in patients given benzodiazepines for even short periods. The symptoms, which may persist for weeks or months, include anxiety, depression, nausea, insomnia and perceptual changes.

Drug interactions. Benzodiazepines have additive or synergistic effects with other central depressants such as alcohol, barbiturates and antihistamines.

Intravenous benzodiazepines (e.g. *diazepam*, *clonazepam*) are used in status epilepticus (Chaper 24) and very occasionally in panic attacks (however, oral *alprazolam* is probably more effective for this latter purpose and is safer). *Midazolam*, unlike other benzodiazepines, forms water-soluble salts and is used as an intravenous sedative during endoscopic and dental procedures.

DRUGS ACTING AT SEROTONERGIC (5HT) RECEPTORS

It is believed that serotonin may be involved in anxiety because, in general, stimulation of this system causes anxiety, whilst a reduction in serotonergic neuronal activity (e.g. by benzodiazepines) reduces anxiety. In the raphe nucleus the dendrites of serotinergic neurones possess inhibitory autoreceptors ($5HT_{1A}$ type) and agonists (e.g. buspirone, gepirone, ipsapirone) acting at this site decrease the firing of 5HT neurones and show anxiolytic properties. *Buspirone* has recently been introduced as an anxiolytic that is non-sedative and seems unlikely to cause dependence. $5HT_{1A}$ agonists may also have antidepressant actions. Another approach to decreasing serotinergic activity in the brain is to block the post-synaptic receptors at the axon terminal synapses. *Ondansetron* is a $5HT_3$ receptor antagonist which probably has anxiolytic properties in addition to its more solidly established antiemetic action (Chapter 40).

β-Adrenoceptor blockers such as propranolol can be very effective in alleviating the autonomic symptoms of anxiety such as tremor, palpitations, sweating and diarrhoea.

Chloral hydrate is converted in the body to trichloroethanol which is an effective hypnotic. It is cheap, but may cause gastric irritation. *Dichloralphenazone* is a derivative of chloral hydrate that is not a gastric irritant. These drugs are useful in the young and elderly. They can cause tolerance and dependence.

Chlormethiazole has no advantage over short-acting benzodiazepines, except in the elderly where it may cause less hangover. It is given by intravenous infusion in acute alcohol withdrawal and in status epilepticus.

Sedative antidepressants such as *amitriptyline* are appropriate if insomnia is associated with depression (Chapter 27).

24 Antiepileptic drugs

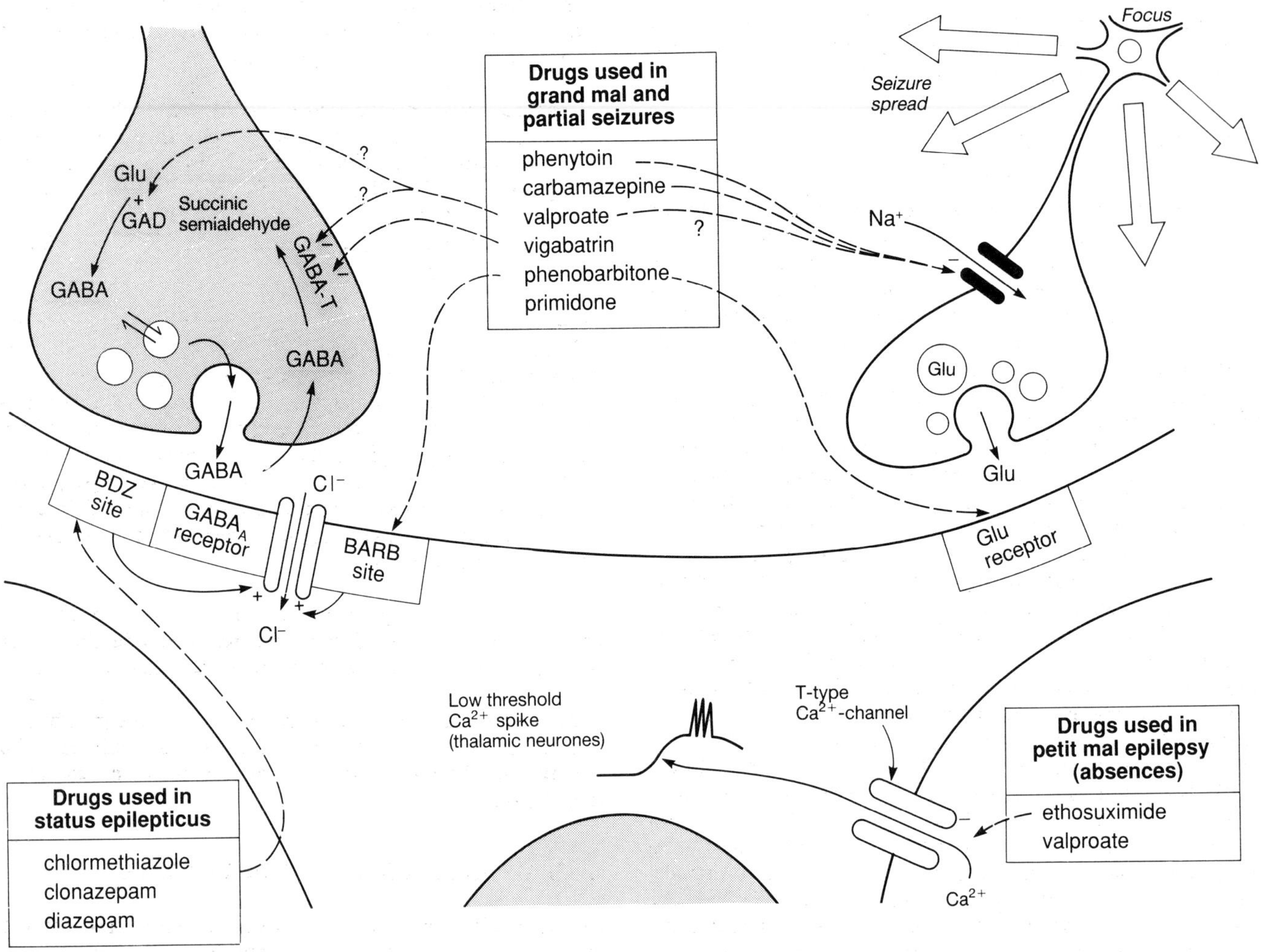

Epilepsy is a chronic disease in which seizures result from the abnormal discharge of cerebral neurones. The seizures are classified empirically.

Partial (focal) seizures begin at a specific locus (upper right figure) in the brain and may be limited to clonic jerking of an extremity. However, the discharge may spread (⇦) and become generalized (**secondarily generalized seizure**). **Generalized seizures** are those in which there is no evidence of localized onset. They include **tonic-clonic** attacks (*grand mal*—periods of tonic rigidity followed later by massive jerking of the body) and **absences** (*petit mal*—changes in consciousness usually lasting less than 10 seconds).

Tonic-clonic and partial seizures are treated mainly with oral **phenytoin** or **carbamazepine** (top middle); the latter agent is usually used for partial seizures and in young females. **Valproate** is an alternative agent. These drugs are of similar effectiveness and a single drug will control the fits in 70–80% of patients with tonic-clonic seizures, but only 30–40% of patients with partial seizures. In these poorly controlled patients, the addition of **vigabatrin** may reduce the incidence of seizures. **Phenobarbitone**, primidone and clonazepam are alternative drugs, but are very sedative.

Absence seizures are usually treated with **ethosuximide** (bottom right), but valproate and clonazepam are alternatives. Petit mal only occasionally continues into adult life, but about 50% of children will later develop grand mal fits.

Status epilepticus is a state in which fits follow each other without consciousness being regained. Urgent treatment with intravenous agents (bottom left) is necessary to stop the fits, which, if unchecked, result in exhaustion and cerebral damage.

Antiepileptic drugs control seizures by mechanisms that are often unclear, but usually involve either the enhancement of GABA-mediated inhibition (benzodiazepines, vigabatrin, phenobarbitone, valproate) (left of figure) or a reduction of Na^+ fluxes (phenytoin, carbamazepine, valproate) (right figure). Ethosuximide may inhibit a spike-generating Ca^{2+} current in thalamic neurones (bottom right).

CAUSES OF EPILEPSY

The aetiology is unknown in 60–70% of cases, but heredity is an important factor. Damage to the brain, for example, tumours, asphyxia, infections or head injury may subsequently cause epilepsy. Convulsions may be precipitated in epileptics by several groups of drugs, including *phenothiazines*, *tricyclic antidepressants* and many *antihistamines*.

MECHANISMS OF ACTION OF ANTICONVULSANTS

The most-studied agent is **phenytoin**, which at therapeutic concentrations has no effect on transmitter release or on neuronal responses to glutamate or GABA. Its anticonvulsant action is probably due to its ability to *prevent high-frequency repetitive activity*. Just how phenytoin does this is not clear, but in voltage clamp experiments, it has been shown to increase the proportion of inactivated Na^+ channels for any given membrane potential. Phenytoin binds preferentially to inactivated (closed) Na^+ channels, stabilizing them in the inactivated state and preventing them from returning to the resting (closed) state that they must re-enter before they can again open (see Chapter 5). High frequency repetitive depolarization increases the proportion of Na^+ channels in the inactivated state and because these are susceptible to blockade by phenytoin, the Na^+ current is progressively reduced until it is eventually insufficient to evoke an action potential. Neuronal transmission at normal frequencies is relatively unaffected by phenytoin, because a much smaller proportion of the Na^+ channels are in the inactivated state. **Carbamazepine** and perhaps **valproate** have similar actions on neuronal Na^+ channels. Valproate also seems to increase GABAergic central inhibition by mechanisms that may involve stimulation of GAD activity and/or inhibition of GABA-T activity. **Vigabatrin** is an irreversible inhibitor of GABA-T which increases brain GABA levels and central GABA release. The benzodiazepines (e.g. **clonazepam**) and **phenobarbitone** also increase central inhibition, but by enhancing the action of synaptically released GABA at the $GABA_A$ receptor/Cl^- channel complex (Chapter 23). Phenobarbitone may also reduce the effects of glutamate at excitatory synapses.

The mechanism of action of **ethosuximide** is unclear. Absence seizures involve oscillatory neuronal activity between the thalamus and cerebral cortex. This oscillation involves (T-type) Ca^{2+} channels in the thalamic neurones, which produce low threshold spikes and allow the cells to fire in bursts. Recent evidence suggests that ethosuximide reduces this Ca^{2+} current, dampening the thalamocortical oscillations that are critical in the generation of absence seizures.

DRUGS USED IN PARTIAL AND GRAND MAL SEIZURES

Phenytoin is hydroxylated in the liver by a saturable enzyme system. The rate of metabolism varies greatly in different patients, and up to 20 days may be required for the serum level to stabilize after changing the dose. Therefore, the dose may be increased gradually until fits are prevented, or until signs of *cerebellar disturbance* occur (nystagmus, ataxia, dysarthria). Measurement of serum drug levels is extremely valuable, because once the metabolizing enzymes are saturated, a small increase in dose may produce toxic blood levels of the drug. *Adverse effects* include drowsiness, cerebellar disturbances and, with prolonged treatment, it may cause gum hypertrophy, acne, greasy skin, coarsening of the facial features and hirsutism (hence its avoidance in young females).

Carbamazepine is metabolized in the liver to carbamazepine-10, 11-epoxide, an active metabolite which partly contributes to both its anticonvulsant action and neurotoxicity. In contrast to phenytoin, there is a linear increase in serum concentration with dosage. Mild neurotoxic effects are common (nausea, headache, drowsiness, diplopia and ataxia) and often determine the limit of dosage.

Barbiturates. Only the long-acting barbiturates are anticonvulsants and **phenobarbitone** is the most widely used. It is probably as effective as carbamazepine and phenytoin in the treatment of tonic-clonic and partial seizures, but it is much more sedative. Tolerance occurs with prolonged use and sudden withdrawal may precipitate status epilepticus. Side-effects include *cerebellar symptoms* (e.g. sedation, ataxia, nystagmus), drowsiness in adults and hyperkinesia in children. **Primidone** is metabolized to active anticonvulsant metabolites, one of which is phenobarbitone.

Vigabatrin is a recently introduced drug. Its only indication at present is as an 'add-on' drug for the treatment of epilepsy that is not satisfactorily controlled by other antiepileptic drugs.

Some anticonvulsants, especially phenytoin, phenobarbitone and carbamazepine are *liver enzyme inducers* and stimulate the metabolism of many drugs, e.g. oral contraceptives, warfarin, theophylline.

DRUGS USED TO TREAT PETIT MAL

Ethosuximide is only effective in the treatment of absences and myoclonic seizures (brief jerky movements without loss of consciousness).

DRUGS EFFECTIVE IN GRAND MAL AND PETIT MAL EPILEPSY

Valproate. The advantages of valproate are its relative lack of sedative effects, its wide spectrum of activity and the mild nature of most of its adverse effects (nausea, weight gain, bleeding tendencies and transient hair loss). The main disadvantage is that occasional idiosyncratic responses cause *severe or fatal hepatic toxicity*.

Benzodiazepines. *Clonazepam* is a potent anticonvulsant that is effective in absences, tonic-clonic seizures and myoclonus. It is very sedative and tolerance occurs with prolonged oral administration. In status epilepticus, intravenous clonazepam or diazepam may be effective, but a continuous infusion of chlormethiazole is the treatment of choice.

25 Drugs used in Parkinsonism

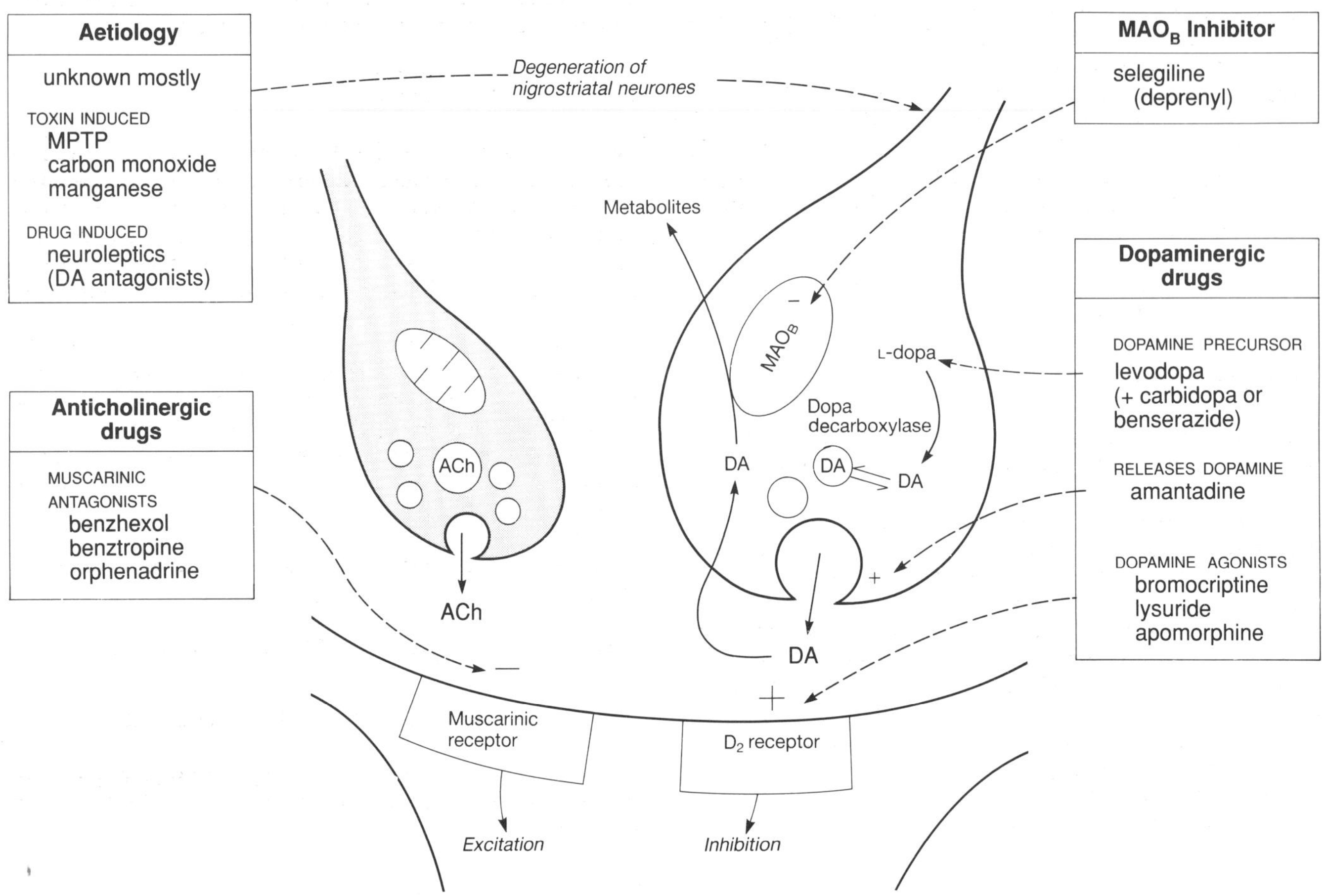

Parkinsonism is a disease of the basal ganglia and is characterized by a poverty of movement, rigidity and tremor. It is progressive and leads to increasing disability unless effective treatment is given.

In the early 1960s, analysis of brains of patients dying with Parkinsonism revealed greatly decreased levels of **dopamine** in the **basal ganglia** (caudate nucleus, putamen, globus pallidus). Parkinsonism thus became the first disease to be associated with a specific transmitter abnormality in the brain. The main pathology in Parkinsonism is extensive degeneration of the dopaminergic **nigrostriatal tract**, but the cause of the degeneration is usually unknown (top left). The cell bodies of this tract are localized in the substantia nigra in the midbrain, and it seems that frank symptoms of Parkinsonism only appear when more than 80% of these neurones have degenerated. About one-third of patients with Parkinsonism eventually develop dementia.

Replacement therapy with dopamine itself is not possible in Parkinsonism because dopamine does not pass the blood–brain barrier. However, its precursor, **levodopa** (L-dopa) does penetrate the brain, where it is decarboxylated to dopamine (right figure). Orally administered levodopa is largely metabolized outside the brain and so it is given with a selective **extracerebral decarboxylase inhibitor** (*carbidopa* or *benserazide*). This greatly decreases the effective dose by reducing peripheral metabolites and reduces peripheral adverse effects (*nausea, postural hypotension*). Levodopa, together with a peripheral decarboxylase inhibitor, is the mainstay of treatment. Other dopaminergic drugs used in Parkinsonism (bottom right) are directly acting **dopamine agonists** and **amantadine**, which causes dopamine release. Some of the peripheral side-effects of dopaminergic drugs can be reduced with *domperidone*, a dopamine antagonist that does not penetrate the brain. Inhibition of monoamine oxidase B (MAO$_B$) with **selegiline** (top right) is ineffective alone, but potentiates the actions of levodopa.

As the nigrostriatal neurones progressively degenerate in Parkinsonism, the release of (inhibitory) dopamine declines and the excitatory cholinergic interneurones in the striatum become relatively 'overactive' (left, ▢). This simple idea provides the rationale for treatment with **anticholinergic agents** (bottom left), but their use in the modern treatment of Parkinsonism is questionable.

AETIOLOGY

The cause of Parkinsonism is unknown and no endogenous or environmental neurotoxin has been discovered. However, the possibility that such a chemical exists has been suggested dramatically by the recent discovery in Californian drug addicts (who were trying to make pethidine) that 1-methyl-4-phenyl-1,2,3,6-tetrahydropyridine (MPTP) causes degeneration of the nigrostriatal tract and Parkinsonism. MPTP acts indirectly via a metabolite, 1-methyl-4-phenylpyridine (MPP^+) which is formed by the action of MAO_B. It is not certain how MPP^+ kills dopaminergic nerve cells, but free radicals generated during its formation by MAO_B may poison mitochondria and/or damage the cell membrane by peroxidation.

Neuroleptic drugs (Chapter 26) block dopamine receptors and often produce a Parkinsonism-like syndrome.

DOPAMINERGIC DRUGS

Levodopa with a selective extracerebral decarboxylase inhibitor is the best treatment for most patients with Parkinsonism.

Mechanism. Levodopa is the immediate precursor of dopamine and is able to penetrate the brain, where it is converted to dopamine. The site of this decarboxylation in the parkinsonian brain is uncertain, but as dopa decarboxylase is not rate-limiting, there may be sufficient enzyme in the remaining dopaminergic nerve terminals. Another possibility is that the conversion occurs in noradrenergic or serotonergic terminals, because the decarboxylase activity in these neurones is not specific. In any event, the release of dopamine replaced in the brain by levodopa therapy must be very abnormal, and it is remarkable that most patients with Parkinsonism benefit, often dramatically, from its administration.

Adverse effects are frequent, and mainly result from widespread stimulation of dopamine receptors. *Nausea* and *vomiting* are caused by stimulation of the chemoreceptor trigger zone in the area postrema, which lies outside the blood–brain barrier. This can be reduced by the peripherally acting dopamine antagonist domperidone. *Psychiatric* side-effects are the most common limiting factor in levodopa treatment and include vivid dreams, hallucinations, psychotic states and confusion. These effects are probably due to stimulation of mesolimbic or mesocortical dopamine receptors (remember overactivity in these systems is associated with schizophrenia). Postural hypotension is common but often asymptomatic. *Dyskinesias* are an important adverse effect that in the early stages of Parkinsonism usually reflect overtreatment and respond to simple dose reduction (or fractionation).

Problems with long-term treatment. After 5 years treatment about half of patients will have lost ground. In some there is a gradual recurrence of parkinsonian akinesia. A second form of deterioration is the shortening of duration of action of each dose of levodopa ('*end-of-dose deterioration*'). Various dyskinesias may appear and, with time, many patients start to get increasingly severe and rapid oscillations in mobility and dyskinesias—the '*on–off' effect*. These fluctuations in response are related to the peaks and troughs of plasma levodopa levels. It seems that progressive neuronal degeneration reduces the capacity of the striatum to buffer fluctuating levodopa levels, because continuous dopaminergic stimulation produced by the intravenous infusion of levodopa, or subcutaneous infusion of apomorphine, control the dyskinesias. Unfortunately, this form of treatment is not generally practical, but a simpler strategy of combining oral levodopa with single injections of apomorphine given during the 'off' periods, helps many advanced fluctuating parkinsonian patients to have a more stable day.

DOPAMINE AGONISTS

Bromocriptine is a selective D_2-agonist. It is often given in combination with levodopa in the later stages of Parkinsonism in an attempt to reduce the late adverse effects of levodopa ('wearing-off' and 'on–off' phenomena). The adverse effects of bromocriptine are similar to those of levodopa (i.e. nausea, psychiatric symptoms, postural hypotension), but are more common and tend to be more severe.

Bromocriptine inhibits the release of prolactin from the pituitary and is used in the treatment of *hyperprolactinaemia*. It is also used to suppress growth hormone release in *acromegaly*, although in normal people, the drug increases hormone release. The suppression of growth hormone in acromegalics occurs because of the presence of dopamine receptors that are not expressed in normal people.

Lysuride is a D_2-agonist with similar actions to bromocriptine, but psychiatric side-effects are more severe.

Apomorphine stimulates D_1 and D_2 dopamine receptors.

DRUGS CAUSING DOPAMINE RELEASE

Amantadine has muscarinic blocking actions and probably increases dopamine release. It has modest anti-parkinsonian effects, but tolerance soon occurs.

MAO_B INHIBITOR

Selegiline (deprenyl) selectively inhibits MAO_B present in the brain, and for which dopamine, but not noradrenaline or serotonin, is a substrate. It reduces the metabolism of dopamine in the brain and potentiates the actions of levodopa, the dose of which can be reduced by up to one-third. The exciting aspect of selegiline is that there is some evidence that it may actually slow the progression of the disease.

ANTICHOLINERGIC AGENTS

Muscarinic antagonists produce a modest improvement, in the early stages of Parkinsonism, but the akinesia which is responsible for most of the functional disability responds least well. Furthermore, adverse effects are common and include dry mouth, urinary retention, constipation and psychiatric effects that range from mild memory loss to acute confused states.

TRANSPLANTATION

Transplantation of nigral cells from human fetuses into the putamen of patients with Parkinsonism have sometimes been rewarded with graft survival and behavioural improvement. However, the role of transplantation in treatment is unlikely to be clear for many years.

26 Drugs used in psychosis—neuroleptics

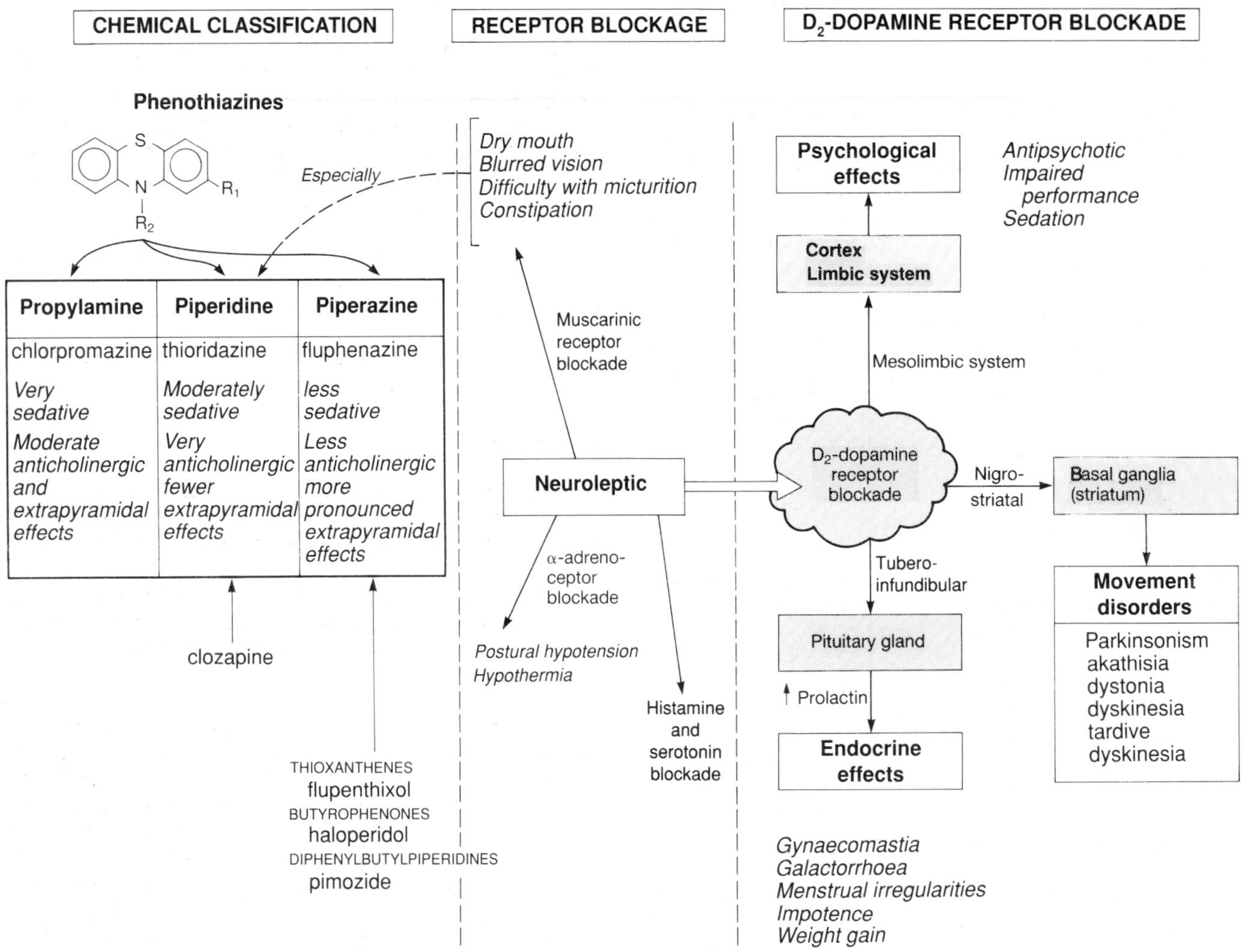

Schizophrenia is a syndrome characterized by specific psychological manifestations. These include auditory hallucinations, delusions, thought disorders and behavioural disturbances. Recent evidence suggests that schizophrenia is probably caused by a genetically determined developmental abnormality which preferentially affects the medial temporal lobe (parahippocampal gyrus, hippocampus and amygdala). Neuroleptic drugs control many of the symptoms of schizophrenia. They have most effect on the positive symptoms such as hallucinations and delusion. Negative symptoms such as social withdrawal and emotional apathy are less affected by neuroleptic drugs. The neuroleptics are all **antagonists at dopamine receptors**, suggesting that schizophrenia is associated with increased activity in the dopaminergic *mesolimbic* and/or *mesocortical pathway* (top right). In agreement with this idea, amphetamine (which causes noradrenaline and dopamine release) can produce a psychotic state in normal subjects, indistinguishable from paranoid schizophrenia. Neuroleptic drugs require several weeks to control the symptoms of schizophrenia and most patients will require maintenance treatment for many years. This may be more readily achieved by the use of **depot preparations**.

Unfortunately, neuroleptics also block dopamine receptors in the basal ganglia (striatum) and this frequently results in distressing and disabling **movement disorders** (right). These include Parkinsonism (which may require treatment with anticholinergic drugs), acute dystonic reactions, akathisia (restlessness and anxiety) and tardive dyskinesia (orofacial and trunk movements) which may be irreversible. It is not known what causes tardive dyskinesia, but because it may be made worse by removing the drug, it has been suggested that the striatal dopamine receptors become supersensitive. Another suggestion is that chronic neuroleptic administration damages striatal GABAergic neurones.

In the pituitary gland, dopamine acting on D_2-dopamine receptors inhibits prolactin release. This effect is blocked by neuroleptics and the resulting increase in prolactin release often causes **endocrine side-effects** (bottom right).

Neuroleptics have **muscarinic receptor** and α-adrenoceptor blocking actions and cause **autonomic side-effects** (middle) including postural hypotension, dry mouth and constipation. The potency of individual drugs in blocking autonomic receptors, and therefore their predominant peripheral side-effects, depends on the **chemical class** to which they belong (left).

DOPAMINE RECEPTORS

In the brain, dopamine receptors have been subdivided, until recently, into two types (D_1 and D_2). Recently, three additional receptors have been cloned and their amino acid sequences determined. The dopamine receptors all display the seven transmembrane-spanning domains characteristic of G-protein-linked receptors.

D_1-dopamine receptors mediate the stimulation of adenylyl cyclase. This stimulation, by dopamine and other dopaminergic agonists, is antagonized by most neuroleptic drugs. However, the antagonist activity of neuroleptics at the D_1-receptor does not correlate with their antipsychotic activity. In particular, the *butyrophenones* are potent neuroleptics, but are weak D_1-receptor antagonists.

D_2-dopamine receptors were identified by binding studies using a radiolabelled butyrophenone, *^{3}H-haloperidol.* D_2-receptors are found in the striatal, limbic and cortical brain regions. Activation of D_2-receptors inhibits adenylyl cyclase activity. The affinity of neuroleptic drugs for the D_2-receptor correlates closely with their antipsychotic potency and this provides circumstantial evidence for the view that schizophrenia is somehow linked to 'overactivity' in a central dopaminergic pathway and that the D_2-receptors are involved.

D_3-dopamine receptors are localized mainly in limbic and cortical structures concerned with cognitive functions and emotional behaviour. Most neuroleptic drugs are 10–20 times more potent at D_2- than D_3-receptors, and because there are high densities of D_2-receptors in the areas of the caudate nucleus that receive fibres from the nigrostriatal tract, extrapyramidal side-effects (movement disorders) are very common. It is not known whether the antipsychotic effects of neuroleptic drugs involve blockade of D_3-receptors as well as D_2-receptors. D_4-dopamine receptors are similar to the D_3-type. Clozapine has a particularly high affinity for the D_4-receptors.

Mechanism of action of neuroleptics. It is not known how neuroleptic drugs reduce the severity of the symptoms in schizophrenia. Since all antipsychotic drugs are dopamine antagonists, it is assumed that schizophrenia is associated with 'overactivity' in the mesolimbic/mesocortical pathways. However, no convincing changes in the dopaminergic system (or any other transmitter system) have been found in schizophrenia.

CHEMICAL CLASSIFICATION

Drugs with a wide variety of structures have antipsychotic activity, but they all have the ability to block dopamine receptors in common. (Reserpine is not a dopamine antagonist but is a neuroleptic, presumably because it depletes the brain of dopamine as well as noradrenaline and serotonin.)

Phenothiazines are subdivided according to the type of side-chain attached to the N-atom of the phenothiazine ring.

1 Propylamine side-chain. Phenothiazines with an aliphatic side-chain are of relatively low potency and produce nearly all of the side-effects shown in the figure. *Chlorpromazine* was the first phenothiazine used in schizophrenia and is widely used, although it produces more adverse effects than newer drugs. It is very sedative and is particularly useful in treating violent patients. Adverse effects include sensitivity reactions such as agranulocytosis, haemolytic anaemia, rashes, cholestatic jaundice and photosensitization.

2 Piperidine side-chain. The main drug in this group is *thioridazine.* The advantage of this drug, which is favoured in the elderly, is that it is relatively rarely associated with movement disorders and does not cause troublesome hangover drowsiness. Anticholinergic activity is marked and it may cause sexual dysfunction, including retrograde ejaculation. Rarely, high doses may cause retinal degeneration.

3 Piperazine side-chain. Drugs in this group are widely used and include *fluphenazine, prochlorperazine, perphenazine* and *trifluoperazine.* These drugs are less sedative and less anticholinergic than chlorpromazine, but are particularly likely to cause movement disorders, especially in the elderly, where thioridazine is preferred.

Other chemical classes

Butyrophenones. **Haloperidol** has little anticholinergic action and is less sedative and hypotensive than chlorpromazine. However, there is a high incidence of movement disorders.

Diphenylbutylpiperidines. **Pimozide** is not sedative and has a more specific action at dopamine receptors than other drugs. This results in fewer peripheral side-effects, but frequent movement disorders.

Atypical drugs (*clozapine, thioridazine*) are so called because they are associated with a lower incidence of movement disorders. The reason for this is not known. It may be significant that the atypical neuroleptics have a relatively high affinity for D_3-dopamine receptors compared with other neuroleptics, but even the atypical drugs are two to three times more potent at D_2-receptors than D_3-receptors. Another possibility is that the high anticholinergic activity of these drugs inhibits the onset of movement disorders. *Clozapine* is a dibenzodiazepine. It is regarded by some as the only truly atypical neuroleptic, because it has been shown in double-blind trials to be effective, sometimes, in patients refractory to other neuroleptic drugs (i.e. about 10–20% of hospital-treated patients) and almost never causes movement disorders. The drug is restricted to this group of refractory patients because it causes potentially fatal agranulocytosis in about 2% of patients. (Blood samples are required every 1–2 weeks to monitor white cells.) Clozapine has high anticholinergic activity, but it may be atypical because it binds strongly to the D_4-receptors which are present in some limbic areas, but are less numerous in the basal ganglia.

DEPOT PREPARATIONS

Schizophrenic patients are increasingly being 'returned to the community'. This has led to an increased use of long-acting depot injections for maintenance therapy. Oily injections of the decanoate derivatives of *flupenthixol, haloperidol* and *fluphenazine* may be given at intervals of 1–4 weeks, but these preparations increase the incidence of movement disorders.

27 Drugs used in affective disorders—antidepressants

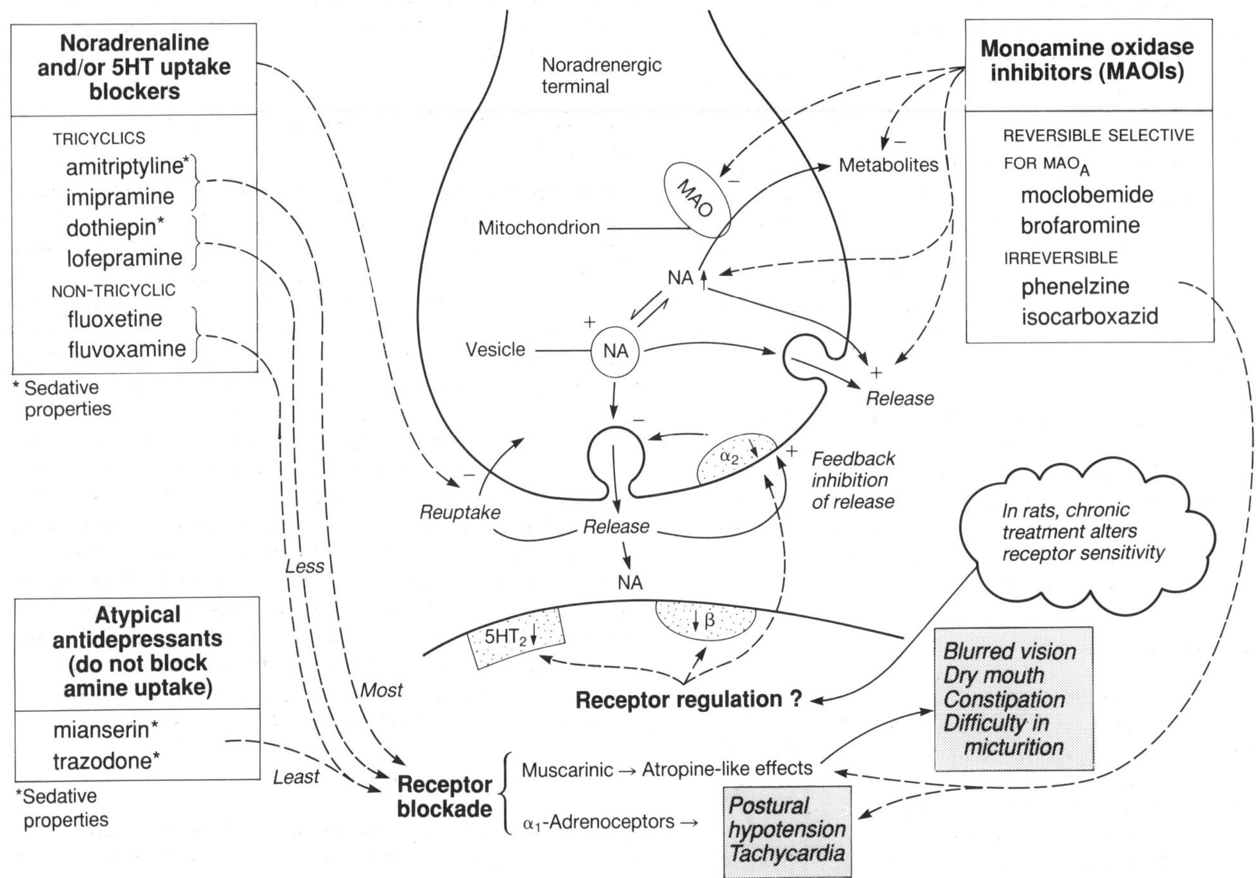

Affective disorders are characterized by a disturbance of mood associated with alterations in behaviour, energy, appetite, sleep and weight. The extremes range from intense excitement and elation **(mania)** to severe **depressive states**. In depression, which is much more common than mania, a person becomes persistently sad and unhappy. Depression is common, and although it can cause people to kill themselves, in general the prognosis is good.

The drugs used most often in the treatment of depression inhibit the uptake of both noradrenaline and 5HT (tricyclics) or are specific inhibitors of 5HT uptake (non-tricyclics) (top left). **Monoamine oxidase inhibitors** (MAOIs) (top right) have been used less often because of dangerous interactions with some foods and drugs. However, the recent introduction of reversible MAOIs (top right) may lead to an increase in the use of this type of drug.

Some 'atypical' drugs are not MAOIs and do not inhibit amine uptake (bottom left). Antidepressant drugs often produce *sedation*, which can be useful, and *autonomic effects* (▢) which are a problem and may be dose-limiting. All antidepressants may provoke seizures and no particular drug is safe for the depressed epileptic patient. A striking characteristic of antidepressant treatment with drugs is that the benefit does not become apparent for 2–3 weeks. The reason for this is unknown, but may be related to gradual changes in the sensitivity of central 5HT adrenoceptors (▢). About 70% of patients respond satisfactorily to treatment with tricyclic (or related) drugs, but in severe or refractive cases of depression, electroconvulsive therapy (ECT) may be required in addition to drugs. In patients who fail to respond to single drugs and/or ECT, some psychiatrists combine tricyclics with MAOIs or lithium. Dangerous interactions can occur with these drug combinations. Abrupt withdrawal of antidepressant drugs, especially MAOIs may cause nausea, vomiting, panic, anxiety and motor restlessness.

The cause of depression and the mechanisms of action of antidepressants are unknown. The **monoamine theory** was based on the idea that depression resulted from a decrease in the activity of central noradrenergic and/or serotonergic systems. There are serious problems with this theory, but it has not been replaced with a better one. More recently, interest has focussed on the effects of antidepressant treatment on **receptor regulation** in the brain.

In *mania* and in *bipolar affective disorders* (where mania alternates with depression) **lithium** has a mood-stabilizing action. Lithium salts have a low therapeutic : toxic ratio and adverse effects are common. *Carbamazepine* also has mood-stabilizing properties and can be used in patients unable to take lithium.

Monoamine theory of depression. *Reserpine*, which depletes the brain of noradrenaline (NA) and serotonin, often causes depression. In contrast, the *tricyclics* and related compounds block the reuptake of NA and/or serotonin and the MAOIs increase their concentration in the brain. Both of these actions increase the amounts of NA and/or serotonin available in the synaptic cleft. These drug effects suggest that depression might be associated with a decrease in brain NA and/or serotonin function. Much effort has gone into trying to find the expected defects in central noradrenergic and serotonergic systems in depressed patients, but these studies have not produced consistent results. There are several problems with the monoamine theory of depression. In particular, it is difficult to understand why the tricyclic drugs rapidly block NA/serotonin uptake but require weeks of administration to achieve an antidepressant effect. Also, some drugs are antidepressant but do not affect amine uptake (e.g. mianserin, trazodone), whilst cocaine blocks uptake but is not antidepressant.

Receptor regulation. Chronic adminstration of antidepressants to rodents gradually decreases the sensitivity of central $5HT_2$ receptors, β_1- and α_2-adrenoceptors (downregulation). Whether similar changes in receptor sensitivity underlie the antidepressant action of drugs in humans is unknown, but chronic antidepressant treatment has been shown to lower the sensitivity of clonidine (an α_2-adrenoceptor agonist).

DRUGS THAT INHIBIT AMINE UPTAKE

The term 'tricyclic drug' originally referred to compounds based on the dibenzazepine (e.g. imipramine) and dibenzocyclohepadiene (e.g. amitriptyline) ring structures. This widely used term is now misleading because many second-generation antidepressants with similar pharmacological properties to the original tricyclics, possess one, two or four rings.

No individual tricyclic drug has superior antidepressant activity and the choice of drug is determined by the most acceptable or desired side-effects. Thus, drugs with sedative actions such as *amitriptyline* and *dothiepin* are more suitable for agitated and anxious patients and, if given at bedtime, will also act as a hypnotic. The tricyclics resemble the phenothiazines in structure and have similar blocking actions at cholinergic *muscarinic receptors*, *α-adrenoreceptors* and *histamine receptors*. These actions frequently cause dry mouth, blurred vision, constipation, urinary retention, tachycardia and postural hypotension. In overdosage, the anticholinergic activity and a quinidine-like action of the tricyclics on the heart may cause arrhythmias and sudden death. They are contraindicated in heart disease.

Fluvoxamine and *fluoxetine* are selective inhibitors of serotonin uptake that have few of the anticholinergic, cardiac and appetite-stimulating effects of many other antidepressants. However, they do cause other side-effects, notably nausea and headache. These more recent drugs are increasingly used.

ATYPICAL ANTIDEPRESSANTS

These drugs have little or no activity on amine uptake. They generally cause fewer autonomic side-effects and because they are less cardiotoxic they are less dangerous in overdosage. *Mianserin* and *trazodone* are sedative antidepressants. Mianserin has α_2-adrenoceptor blocking activity and by blocking inhibitory α_2-autoreceptors on central noradrenergic nerve endings, it may increase the amount of NA in the synaptic cleft. Mianserin may cause agranulocytosis and aplastic anaemia (particularly in the elderly). Trazodone has no α_2-blocking action, but may cause postural hypotension and, less commonly, priapism (a painful and embarrassing state of persistent penile erection).

MONOAMINE OXIDASE INHIBITORS (MAOIs)

The established MAOIs (e.g. *phenelzine*) are irreversible non-selective inhibitors of MAO and appear to be most useful in atypical depression and phobic anxiety states. Their usefulness is limited by adverse effects (postural hypotension, dizziness, anticholinergic effects and liver damage) and by interactions with sympathomimetic amines (e.g. *ephedrine*, often present in cough mixtures and decongestive preparations), or foods containing *tyramine* (e.g. cheese, game, alcoholic drinks) which may result in severe hypertension. Ingested tyramine is normally metabolized by MAO in the gut wall and liver, but when the enzyme is inhibited, tyramine reaches the circulation and causes the release of noradrenaline from sympathetic nerve endings (indirect sympathomimetic action). Monoamine oxidase inhibitors are not specific and reduce the metabolism of barbiturates, opioid analgesics and alcohol. Pethidine is especially dangerous in patients taking MAOIs, causing (by an unknown mechanism) hyperpyrexia, hypotension and coma. Recently developed MAOIs (e.g. *moclobemide*) which are reversible and selective for MAO_A are much safer than the previous drugs and appear to have few adverse effects.

LITHIUM

Lithium is used for prophylaxis in *manic/depressive* illness. It is also used in the treatment of *acute mania*, but, because it lacks marked sedative properties, **neuroleptics** are usually preferred for acutely disturbed patients.

Lithium is rapidly absorbed from the gut. The therapeutic and toxic doses are similar and serum lithium concentrations must be measured regularly (therapeutic range 0.5–1.0 mM). Adverse effects include nausea, vomiting, anorexia, diarrhoea, tremor of the hands, polydipsia and polyuria (a few patients develop nephrogenic diabetes insipidus), hypothyroidism and weight gain. Signs of *lithium toxicity* include drowsiness, ataxia and confusion, and at serum levels above 2–3 mM, life-threatening seizures and coma may occur.

Mechanism of action. This is unknown, but much current interest is focussed on interactions with second-messenger systems. In particular, lithium at concentrations of less than 1 mM blocks the phosphatidylinositol (PI) pathway at the point where inositol-1-phosphate is hydrolysed to inositol. This causes depletion of membrane PIP_2 (see Chapter 1) and may reduce the actions of transmitters acting at receptors which involve inositol triphosphate/diacylglycerol (IP_3/DG) as their second messengers. The selectivity of lithium might be because the blood–brain barrier prevents the entry of myoinositol into the brain. Thus, the inhibition by lithium of myoinositol recycling into phosphoinositides affects phosphoinositides in the brain much more than in peripheral tissues.

28 Opioid analgesics

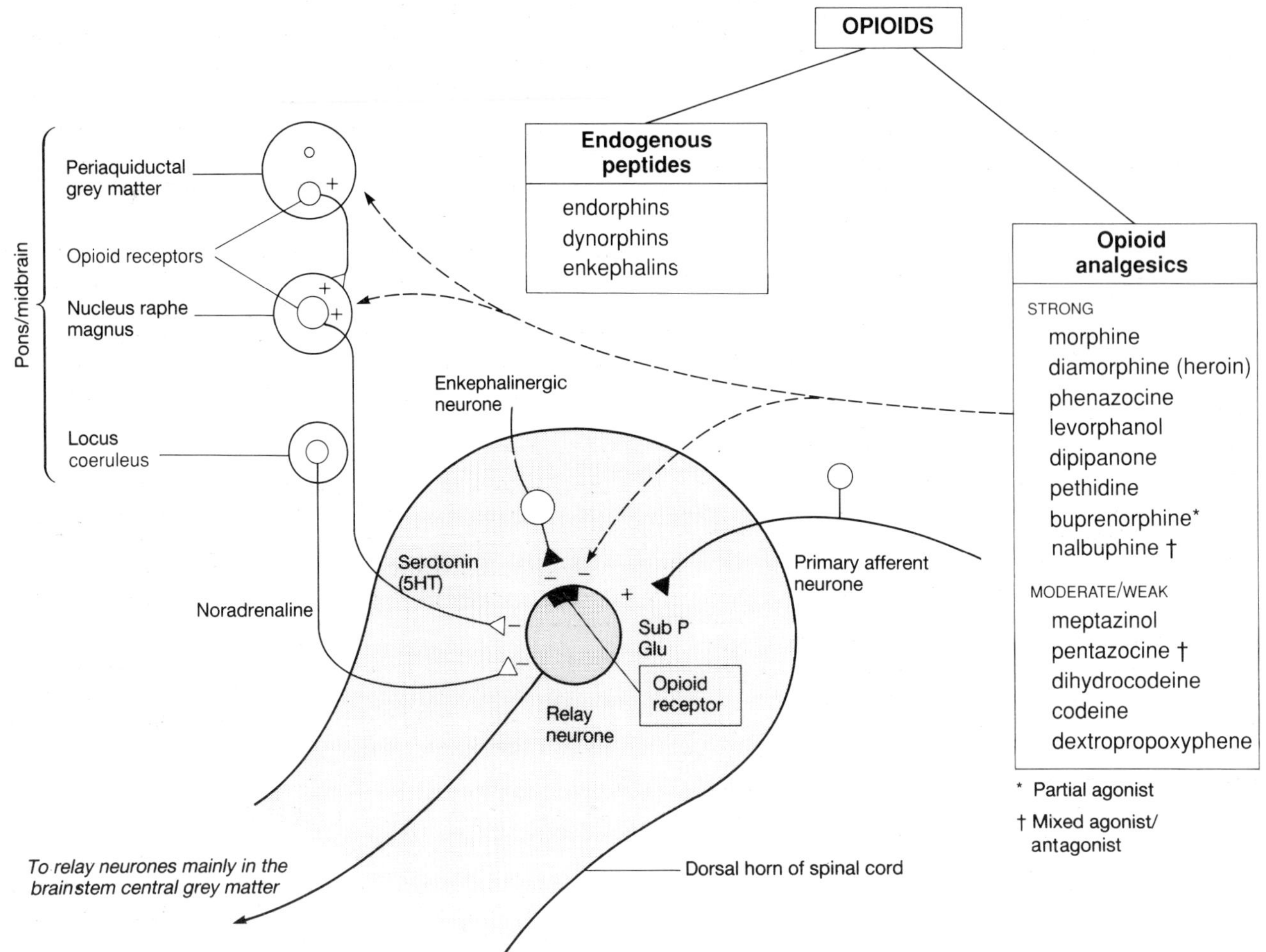

Pain receptors, when stimulated by noxious stimuli, initiate firing in primary afferent fibres which synapse in lamina I and II of the dorsal horn of the spinal cord. The relay neurones (●) in the dorsal horn transmit pain information to the sensory cortex via neurones in the brainstem. Little is known about the transmitter substances utilized in the ascending pain pathways, but some primary afferent fibres are thought to release peptides (e.g. *substance P*, *calcitonin gene-related peptides*, *bradykinin*) (lower figure, shaded).

The activity of the dorsal horn relay neurones is modulated by several *inhibitory inputs*. These include local interneurones which release **opioid peptides** (e.g. [Met^5]enkephalin, dynorphin A) and descending *noradrenergic* and *serotonergic* fibres which originate in the brainstem (top left) and are themselves activated by *opioid peptides*. Thus, opioid peptide release in both the brainstem and the spinal cord can *reduce* the activity of the dorsal horn relay neurones and can cause analgesia. How the different inhibitory mechanisms are normally controlled is unknown, but the effects of opioid peptides are mediated by specific **opioid receptors**.

Opioid analgesics (right) are drugs which mimic endogenous opioid peptides by causing a prolonged activation of opioid receptors. This produces analgesia, respiratory depression, euphoria and sedation. Opioids often cause nausea and vomiting and antiemetics may be required. Effects on the nerve plexuses in the gut, which also possess opioid peptides and receptors, causes constipation and laxatives are usually required (Chapter 13). Continuous treatment with opioid analgesics results in **tolerance** and **dependence** in addicts. However, in terminally ill patients, a steady increase in morphine dosage is not automatic, and where it does occur, is more likely to result from progressively increasing pain rather than tolerance. Similarly, in the clinical context, dependence is unimportant. *Unfortunately, overcaution in the use of opioid analgesics frequently results in unnecessarily poor pain control in patients.*

Some analgesics, such as **codeine**, are less potent than morphine and cannot be given in equianalgesic doses because of the onset of adverse effects. As a result of this restriction in dosage, they are less likely, in practice, to produce respiratory depression and dependence. They are useful in mild to moderate pain.

Naloxone is a specific antagonist at opioid receptors and reverses respiratory depression caused by morphine-like drugs. It also precipitates a withdrawal syndrome when dependence has occurred. Electroacupuncture analgesia, transcutaneous nerve stimulation-induced analgesia and placebo effects can sometimes be partially blocked by naloxone, suggesting the involvement of the endogenous opioid peptides.

Opioids are compounds with effects which are antagonized by naloxone in a stereospecific manner.

There are three families of **opioid peptides** which are derived from large precursor molecules, encoded for by separate genes. All opioid peptides contain the sequence Tyr-Gly-Gly-Phe-Met ([Met^5]enkephalin) or Tyr-Gly-Gly-Phe-Leu ([Leu^5]enkephalin) at their amino terminal. *Pro-opiomelanocortin* (POMC) gives rise to the opioid peptide β-endorphin (31 amino acids) and a number of other non-opioid peptides, including adrenocorticotrophic hormone (ACTH, 39 amino acids). *Proenkephalin* gives rise to [Leu^5]enkephalin, [Met^5]enkephalin and a number of extended [Met^5]enkephalin peptides. *Prodynorphin* gives rise to a number of opioid peptides which contain [Leu^5]enkephalin at their amino terminal (e.g. dynorphin A, 17 amino acids). The peptides derived from each of these three precursor molecules have a distinct anatomical distribution in the central nervous system and have varying affinity for the different types of opioid receptors. The precise function of these opioid peptides in the brain and elsewhere is still unclear.

Opioid receptors are widely distributed throughout the central nervous system and have been classified into three types. The μ-receptors are most highly concentrated in brain areas involved in nociception and are the receptors with which morphine-like drugs interact to produce analgesia. The δ- and κ-receptors display selectivity for the enkephalins and the dynorphins, respectively. The opioid peptides have inhibitory actions on synapses in the central nervous system and gut. Activation of μ- and δ-receptors causes hyperpolarization of neurones by activating K^+ channels by a process involving a G-protein. Activation of κ-receptors inhibits membrane Ca^{2+} channels. Drug action at all three receptors is antagonized by *naloxone*, with increasing doses being required to antagonize actions at μ-, δ- and κ-receptors. Some opioid analgesics (e.g. *pentazocine*) produce stimulant and psychotomimetic effects by acting on σ-receptors and phencyclidine (PCP) receptors. Neither of these receptors are opioid receptors, since these effects are not blocked by naloxone.

STRONG OPIOID ANALGESICS

These are used particularly in the treatment of dull, poorly localized (visceral) pain. Somatic pain is sharply defined and may be relieved by a weak opioid analgesic or by a non-steroidal anti-inflammatory drug (Chapter 30). Parenteral morphine is widely used to treat severe pain and oral morphine is the drug of choice in terminal care.

Morphine and other opioid analgesics produce a range of central effects that include analgesia, euphoria, sedation, respiratory depression, depression of the vasomotor centre (causing postural hypotension), miosis because of IIIrd nerve nucleus stimulation (except pethidine which has weak atropine-like activity) and nausea and vomiting due to stimulation of the chemoreceptor trigger zone. They also cause cough suppression, but this is not correlated with their opioid activity. Peripheral effects include constipation, biliary spasm and constriction of the sphincter of Oddi may occur. Morphine may cause histamine release with vasodilatation and itching. Morphine is metabolized in the liver by conjugation with glucuronic acid to form morphine-3-glucuronide which is inactive, and morphine-6-glucuronide which is a potent analgesic, especially when given intrathecally.

Tolerance (i.e. a decreased responsiveness) to many of the effects of opioid analgesics occurs with continuous administration. Miosis and constipation are effects to which little tolerance develops.

Dependence. Both physical and psychological dependence on opioid analgesics gradually develops and sudden termination of drug administration precipitates a withdrawal syndrome (Chapter 29).

Diamorphine (heroin, diacetylmorphine) is twice as potent as morphine, but is rapidly metabolized to 6-acetylmorphine and more slowly to morphine. It causes more euphoria but relatively less nausea, constipation and hypotension than morphine.

Phenazocine has a more prolonged action than morphine. It is especially useful in biliary colic because it has less effect on biliary pressure than other opioid analgesics.

Pethidine is similar to morphine. Equianalgesic doses depress respiration equally, but it is a poor antitussive and is less constipating. Pethidine is more lipid-soluble than morphine, giving it a rapid onset of action which makes it the drug of choice in labour. Pethidine is metabolized in the liver and at high doses norpethidine can accumulate; this has excitatory actions (dilated pupil, convulsions). Pethidine interacts seriously with MAOIs (Chapter 27) causing delirium, hyperpyrexia and convulsions or respiratory depression.

Buprenorphine is a partial agonist at μ-receptors. It is very lipid-soluble and is an effective analgesic following sublingual administration, but may cause prolonged vomiting. Respiratory depression, if it occurs, is difficult to reverse with naloxone, because buprenorphine dissociates very slowly from the receptors.

Nalbuphine is a κ-agonist and a μ-antagonist which is equipotent with morphine in producing analgesia and respiratory depression, but produces less nausea and vomiting. At higher doses it causes dysphoria.

WEAK OPIOID ANALGESICS

Weak opioid analgesics are used in 'mild to moderate' pain. They may cause dependence and are subject to abuse. However, they are less attractive to addicts because they do not give a good 'buzz'.

Pentazocine is an unpleasant weak analgesic orally, but when given by injection its efficacy is somewhere between that of morphine and codeine. It is an agonist at κ- and σ-receptors, but an antagonist at μ-receptors. It is less likely to cause dependence. This may be partly due to the frequency with which it causes hallucinations, bad dreams and thought disorders due to activation of σ-receptors.

Meptazinol is a weak opioid. It causes nausea and vomiting, but is claimed to have a low incidence of respiratory depression.

Codeine (methylmorphine) has about one-twelfth the analgesic potency of morphine, but side-effects (constipation, vomiting, sedation) limit the possible dosage to levels that produce much less analgesia than morphine. Codeine is also used as an antitussive and antidiarrhoeal agent.

Dihydrocodeine is similar to codeine. It may cause dizziness and constipation.

Dextropropoxyphene is about half as potent as codeine, but has similar actions at equianalgesic doses. It is more effective when combined with aspirin or paracetamol (e.g. 'Distalgesic'), but such mixtures are dangerous in overdose. The dextropropoxyphene causes respiratory depression and acute heart failure, whilst the paracetamol is hepatotoxic.

29 Drug misuse and dependence

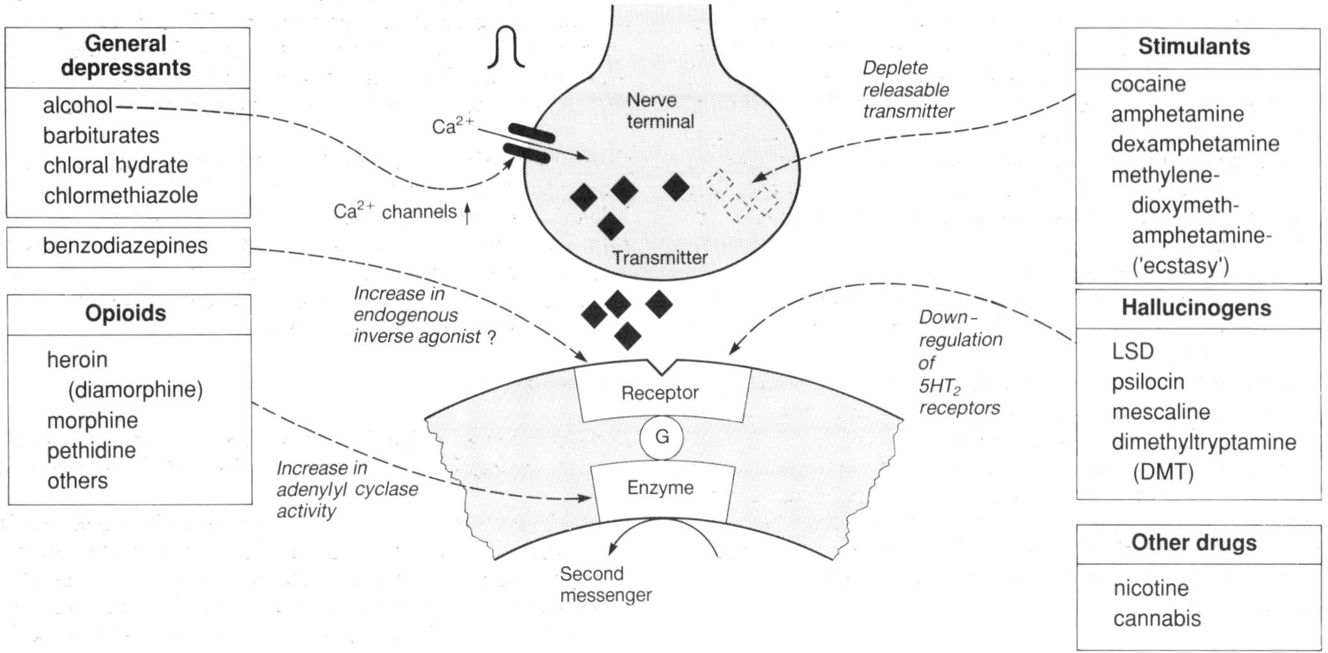

The relationship between drugs that act on the mind and society is one of an uneasy and changing coexistence. For example, there is much popular concern today about the illicit use of opioids, but in the nineteenth century, laudenum, an alcoholic solution of opium, was a popular and readily available home medication. Society now accepts only **alcohol** and **nicotine** (tobacco) as legal psychoactive drugs, although their misuse is responsible for considerable morbidity and mortality. Tobacco consumption alone causes 100 000 deaths each year in Britain.

The term **drug misuse** is applied to any drug taking which harms or threatens to harm the physical or mental health of an individual, or of other individuals, or which is illegal. Thus, drug misuse includes *alcohol* and *nicotine* and the deleterious over-prescription of medicines (e.g. *benzodiazepines*, *stimulants*), as well as the more obvious taking of illicit drugs.

Drug dependence is a term used when a person has a compulsion to take a drug in order to experience its psychic effects, and sometimes to avoid the discomfort of withdrawal symptoms.

The likelihood of drug misuse leading to dependence depends on many factors including the *type of drug*, the *route of administration*, the *pattern of drug taking* and the *individual*. Rapid delivery systems (i.e. intravenous injection, smoking cocaine or heroin) increase the dependence potential. Intravenous injections have attendant dangers of infection (AIDS, hepatitis, septicaemia, etc.).

Drug dependence is often associated with **tolerance**, a phenomenon that may occur with chronic adminstration of a drug. It is characterized by the necessity to progressively increase the dose of the drug to produce its original effect. Tolerance may be due, in part, to increased metabolism of the drug (pharmacokinetic tolerance), but it is mainly caused by neuroadaptive changes in the brain.

The mechanisms underlying drug dependence and tolerance are poorly understood. In general, chronic drug administration induces homeostatic adaptive changes in the brain that operate in a manner to oppose the action of the drug. Withdrawal of the drug causes a rebound in central excitability. Thus, the withdrawal of depressants (e.g. alcohol, barbiturates) may result in convulsions, whilst the withdrawal of excitatory drugs (e.g. amphetamine) results in depression.

Many neuroadaptive changes in the brain have been described following chronic drug administration. They include an increase in Ca^{2+} channels (top left), depletion of transmitter (top right), receptor downregulation (middle right), changes in second messenger (bottom left) and the synthesis of an inverse agonist (middle left).

Central stimulants. *Amphetamine-like* drugs given orally decrease appetite, give a sense of increased energy and well-being and enhance physical performance. They also have peripheral sympathomimetic effects (e.g. hypertension, tachycardia) and cause insomnia. Amphetamine-like drugs cause dopamine and noradrenaline release from nerve terminals, but their behavioural effects are due mainly to dopamine release. *Cocaine* blocks the reuptake of dopamine into nerve terminals and has very similar effects to amphetamine. Stimulants produce dependence because they increase dopaminergic activity in a *reward system* that originates in the *ventral tegmental area* and projects to the *nucleus accumbens* and *frontal cortex*. Thus, the stimulants, and perhaps some other drugs of dependence, act as '*reinforcers*'.

Central stimulants have few indications. They *should not be used as appetite suppressants* in the treatment of obesity, because they do not improve the long-term outlook and often result in dependence.

Cocaine hydrochloride is usually 'snorted' up the nose, but the free base ('crack'), which is more volatile, can be smoked, whereupon it is rapidly absorbed through the lungs and produces a sudden, brief, but overwhelming sense of euphoria ('rush'). A similar 'rush' is produced by intravenous amphetamine, and addicts cannot distinguish between them. The stimulants are highly addictive and are psychotoxic. Repeated administration may produce a state resembling an acute attack of schizophrenia.

Methylenedioxymethamphetamine (MDMA, 'ecstasy') is an amphetamine derivative with mixed stimulant and hallucinogenic properties, the latter action perhaps resulting from 5HT release. MDMA is widely abused as a 'recreational' drug, but it may produce psychiatric illness and occasionally severe acute hyperthermic reactions result in death.

Opioids. Diamorphine (*heroin*) and other opioids have a high misuse and dependence potential because of the intense sense of euphoria they produce when taken intravenously. Tolerance develops quickly in addicts and abrupt withdrawal of opioids results in a craving to take the drug, together with a withdrawal syndrome characterized by yawning, sweating, gooseflesh, tremor, irritability, anorexia, nausea and vomiting, which lasts 7–10 days. Withdrawal of longer-acting drugs such as *methadone* results in a more prolonged, but less intense, syndrome and the treatment of opioid withdrawal usually involves substitution with methadone followed by a slow 'tapering off'. *Clonidine* can suppress some components of the withdrawal syndrome, especially the nausea, vomiting and diarrhoea.

The mechanisms underlying opioid dependence and tolerance are unknown. Chronic administration does not affect opioid receptors, but changes in second messengers may be important; e.g. in the *locus coeruleus*, μ-receptor activation inhibits adenylyl cyclase activity, but with chronic opioid administration the activity of the enzyme increases. Withdrawal of the inhibitory opioid then results in excessive cAMP production, which may contribute to the rebound (increase) of neuronal excitability.

Hallucinogens (*psychedelics*). *Lysergic acid diethylamide* (*LSD*) and related drugs induce dramatic states of altered perception, vivid and unusual sensory experiences and feelings of ecstasy. Occasionally, LSD produces unwanted effects which include panic, frightening delusions and hallucinations. Usually the 'bad trip' fades away, but sometimes it returns later ('flashbacks').

Serotinergic systems may be important in the actions of LSD, which inhibits the firing of 5HT-containing neurones in the *raphe nuclei*, probably by stimulating $5HT_2$ inhibitory autoreceptors on these cells. Tolerance to LSD and related compounds occurs, and is associated with a downregulation of $5HT_2$ receptors. However, physical dependence to hallucinogens does not occur and there is no withdrawal syndrome.

Cannabis (*marijuana, hashish*). The main active constituent of cannabis is Δ'-tetrahydrocannabinol (THC). Cannabis has both hallucinogenic and depressant actions. It produces feelings of euphoria, relaxation and well-being. Cannabis is not dangerously addictive, but at least mild degrees of dependence may occur. Cannabis may cause acute psychotoxic effects that in some ways resemble an LSD 'bad trip'.

General depressants

Barbiturates have a high dependence potential and withdrawal can cause epileptic fits or a state resembling delirium tremens.

Alcohol has effects that resemble those of general anaesthetics. It inhibits presynaptic Ca^{2+} entry (and hence transmitter release) and potentiates GABA-mediated inhibition. Considerable tolerance occurs to alcohol, but the mechanisms involved are poorly understood. Presynaptic Ca^{2+} channels may increase in number, so that when alcohol is withdrawn, transmitter release is abnormally high and this may contribute to the withdrawal syndrome.

Chronic heavy drinking leads to physical dependence and in the United Kingdom there are about 14 800 patients admitted each year to psychiatric hospitals for alcohol dependence and psychosis; brain damage and liver disease leading to cirrhosis are also common.

The physical withdrawal syndromes in humans ranges from a '*hangover*' to *epileptic fits* and the condition of '*delirium tremens*' in which the subject becomes agitated, confused and may have severe hallucinations. Alcohol (and barbiturate) withdrawal may require *chlormethiazole* or *benzodiazepine* administration to prevent convulsions. *Clonidine* may be helpful.

Tobacco (nicotine) is a highly addictive drug that is responsible for more damage to health in the United Kingdom than all other drugs (including alcohol) combined. Nicotine increases alertness, decreases irritability and decreases skeletal muscle tone (because Renshaw cells are stimulated). Tolerance occurs to some effects of nicotine, notably the nausea and vomiting seen in non-tolerant subjects. The *toxicity of tobacco* is due to the many chemicals in the smoke, some of which are known carcinogens. Serious diseases associated with chronic tobacco smoking include lung cancer, coronary heart disease and peripheral vascular disease. Smoking during pregnancy significantly reduces the birth weight of babies and increases perinatal mortality.

Withdrawal of tobacco may cause a syndrome (lasting 2–3 weeks) which includes 'craving' for tobacco, irritability, difficulty in concentration and often weight gain. These symptoms may be reduced by the use of *nicotine chewing gum*. Unfortunately, the craving for tobacco leads to relapse in most people who try to give up smoking, even after myocardial infarction.

30 Non-steroidal anti-inflammatory drugs (NSAIDs)

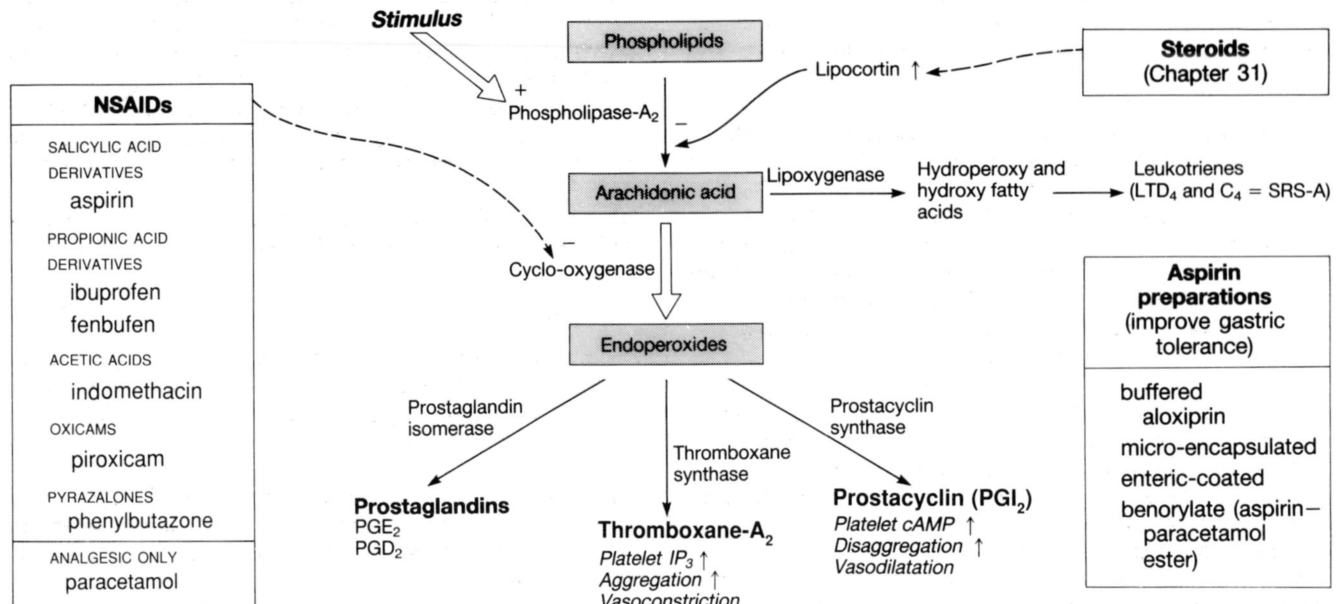

These drugs have in various degrees *analgesic*, *anti-inflammatory* and *antipyretic* actions. They are extensively used and in the United Kingdom almost a quarter of patients consulting their general practitioners have some form of 'rheumatic' complaint. These patients are frequently prescribed NSAIDs and additional millions of aspirin, paracetamol and ibuprofen tablets are bought over the counter for the self-treatment of headaches, dental pain, various musculoskeletal disorders, etc. The large market for NSAIDs has resulted in the steady introduction of new drugs, some of which have proved unacceptably toxic and have been withdrawn.

The NSAIDs form a chemically diverse group (left), but they all have the ability to **inhibit cyclo-oxygenase** (⇨) and the resulting inhibition of prostaglandin synthesis is largely responsible for their therapeutic effects. Unfortunately, the inhibition of prostaglandin synthesis in the gastric mucosa frequently results in *gastrointestinal damage* (dyspepsia, nausea, gastritis and diarrhoea). More serious adverse effects include gastrointestinal bleeding and perforation.

Aspirin (acetylsalicylic acid) is the longest-standing NSAID and is an effective analgesic, with a duration of action of about 4 hours. Aspirin remains the drug of choice for many sorts of mild to moderate pain and certain types of severe pain (e.g. bone cancer). It is not effective in the treatment of visceral pain (e.g. myocardial infarction, renal colic, acute abdomen) which requires narcotic analgesics. Aspirin is well absorbed orally. As it is a weak acid ($pK_a = 3.5$), the acid pH of the stomach keeps a large fraction of aspirin non-ionized and therefore promotes absorption in the stomach, although much aspirin is absorbed via the large surface area of the upper small intestine. The absorbed aspirin is hydrolysed by esterases in the blood and tissues to salicylate (which is active) and acetic acid. Most salicylate is converted in the liver to water-soluble conjugates that are rapidly excreted by the kidney. Alkalinization of the urine ionizes the salicylate and, because this reduces its tubular reabsorption, excretion is increased.

Aspirin is a well-established drug in the treatment of inflammatory joint disease, but up to 50% of patients will not tolerate the adverse effects (nausea, vomiting, epigastric pain, tinnitis) caused by the high doses of soluble aspirin necessary to achieve an anti-inflammatory effect. Various preparations (bottom right) containing aspirin are designed to minimize its gastrointestinal effects, but for treating the symptoms of inflammatory joint disease (pain, stiffness and swelling) newer NSAIDs are generally preferred. Surprisingly few clinical trials have attempted to rank the efficacy of different NSAIDs and most drugs are presently considered to have similar effectiveness. However, there is considerable patient variation in response and so it is impossible to know which drug will be effective in an individual, although 60% of patients will respond to any drug. Since the propionic acid derivatives (e.g. **ibuprofen**) seem to be associated with fewer serious adverse effects, these are often tried first. **Indomethacin** may be effective when other drugs fail, but is associated with a higher incidence of adverse effects.

Paracetamol has no significant anti-inflammatory action, but is widely used as a mild analgesic when pain has no inflammatory component. It is well absorbed orally and does not cause gastric irritation. It has the disadvantage that, in overdosage, serious hepatotoxicity is likely to occur (Chapter 4).

Analgesic action. The analgesic action of NSAIDs is exerted both peripherally and centrally, but the peripheral actions predominate. Their analgesic action is usually associated with their anti-inflammatory action and results from the inhibition of prostaglandin synthesis in the inflamed tissues. Prostaglandins produce little pain by themselves, but potentiate the pain caused by other mediators of inflammation (e.g. histamine, bradykinin).

Anti-inflammatory action. The role of prostaglandins in inflammation is to produce vasodilatation and increased vascular permeability. However, inhibition of prostaglandin synthesis by NSAIDs attenuates rather than abolishes inflammation, because the drugs do not inhibit other mediators of inflammation. Nevertheless, the relatively modest anti-inflammatory actions of the NSAIDs give, to most patients with rheumatoid arthritis, some relief from pain, stiffness, and swelling, but they do not alter the course of the disease.

Antipyretic action. NSAIDs do not reduce the normal body temperature or the elevated temperatures in heat stroke, which is due to hypothalamic malfunction. During fever, endogenous pyrogen (interleukin-1) is released from leucocytes and acts directly on the thermoregulatory centre in the hypothalamus to increase body temperature. This effect is associated with a rise in brain prostaglandins (which are pyrogenic). Aspirin prevents the temperature-raising effects of interleukin-1 and the rise in brain prostaglandin levels.

Mechanism of action on cyclo-oxygenase. NSAIDs inhibit cyclo-oxygenase by several mechanisms. *Aspirin* binds covalently with a serine residue of the enzyme, causing irreversible inhibition. This results from steric hindrance of access of substrate to the oxygenase active site. In contast, *ibuprofen* and *piroxicam* are reversible competitive inhibitors of cyclo-oxygenase. *Paracetamol* acts at least partly by reducing cytoplasmic peroxide tone: peroxide is necessary to activate the haem enzyme to the ferryl form. In areas of acute inflammation, paracetamol is not very effective because neutrophils and monocytes produce high levels of H_2O_2 and lipid peroxide, which overcome the actions of the drug. However, paracetamol is an effective analgesic in conditions where leucocyte infiltration is absent or low.

Adverse effects of NSAIDs are common, partly because the drugs may be given in high doses for a long time and partly because they are widely used in elderly patients who are more susceptible to side-effects.

Gastrointestinal tract. Damage to the mucosa of the gastrointestinal tract seems to be mainly a consequence of prostaglandin synthesis inhibition, rather than a directly erosive action of the drugs. Prostaglandins (PGE_2 and PGI_2) inhibit gastric acid secretion, increase blood flow though the gastric mucosa and have a cytoprotective action (PGE_2 and some analogues induce healing in peptic ulcer). By inhibiting prostaglandin formation, NSAIDs may cause ulceration by producing mucosal ischaemia and by impairing the protective mucus barrier, thus exposing the mucosa to the damaging effects of acid. *Misoprostol* is a PGE_2 derivative that is effective in preventing the gastrointestinal toxicity of NSAIDs. Its main indication is in patients with a history of peptic ulcer whose need for NSAID treatment is such that the analgesic cannot be withdrawn.

Nephrotoxicity. Prostaglandins PGE_2 and PGI_2 are powerful vasodilators synthesized in the renal medulla and glomeruli respectively, and are involved in the control of renal blood flow and excretion of salt and water. Inhibition of renal prostaglandin synthesis may result in sodium retention, reduced renal blood flow and renal failure, especially in patients with conditions associated with vasoconstrictor catecholamine and angiotensin II release (e.g. congestive heart failure, cirrhosis). In addition, NSAIDs may cause interstitial nephritis and hyperkalaemia. Prolonged analgesic abuse over a period of years is associated with papillary necrosis and chronic renal failure.

Other adverse effects include bronchospasm, especially in asthmatics, skin rashes and other allergies.

OTHER NSAIDs

Propionic acids such as *ibuprofen*, *fenbufen* and *naproxen* are widely regarded as the drugs of first choice for the treatment of inflammatory joint disease, because they have the lowest incidence of side-effects.

Acetic acids. *Indomethacin* is one of the more effective agents, but has a high incidence of adverse effects including ulceration, gastric bleeding, headaches and dizziness. It may also cause blood dyscrasias.

Oxicams. *Piroxicam* is an extensively used and potent anti-inflammatory drug. Its main advantage is that it only requires a single daily dose. It may be associated with a particularly high incidence of gastrointestinal bleeding in the elderly.

Pyrazolones. *Phenylbutazone* is an extremely potent anti-inflammatory agent, but has serious toxicity. It is restricted to hospital use for the treatment of intractable pain due to inflammatory arthritis such as ankylosing spondylitis because it sometimes causes fatal aplastic anaemia. *Azapropazone* does not cause bone marrow suppression; it is uricosuric which makes it useful in the management of gouty arthritis.

GOUT

Gout is characterized by deposition of sodium urate crystals in the joint, causing painful arthritis. **Acute attacks** are treated with *indomethacin, naproxen, piroxicam* or other NSAIDs but *not with aspirin*, which raises plasma urate levels at low doses by inhibiting uric acid secretion in the renal tubules. *Colchicine* is effective in gout. It binds to tubulin in leucocytes and prevents their migration to the areas of uric acid deposition and hence reduces the inflammatory responses. However, colchicine causes nausea, vomiting, diarrhoea and abdominal pain.

Prophylactic treatment of gout

Allopurinol lowers plasma urate by inhibiting xanthine oxidase, the enzyme responsible for urate synthesis. It is useful in patients with recurrent attacks of gout.

Uricosuric drugs such as *sulphinpyrazone* and *probenecid* inhibit renal tubular reabsorption of uric acid, increasing its excretion. Plenty of water should be taken to avoid the crystallization of urate in the urine. These drugs are less effective and more toxic than allopurinol. They are normally used in patients who cannot tolerate allopurinol.

31 Corticosteroids

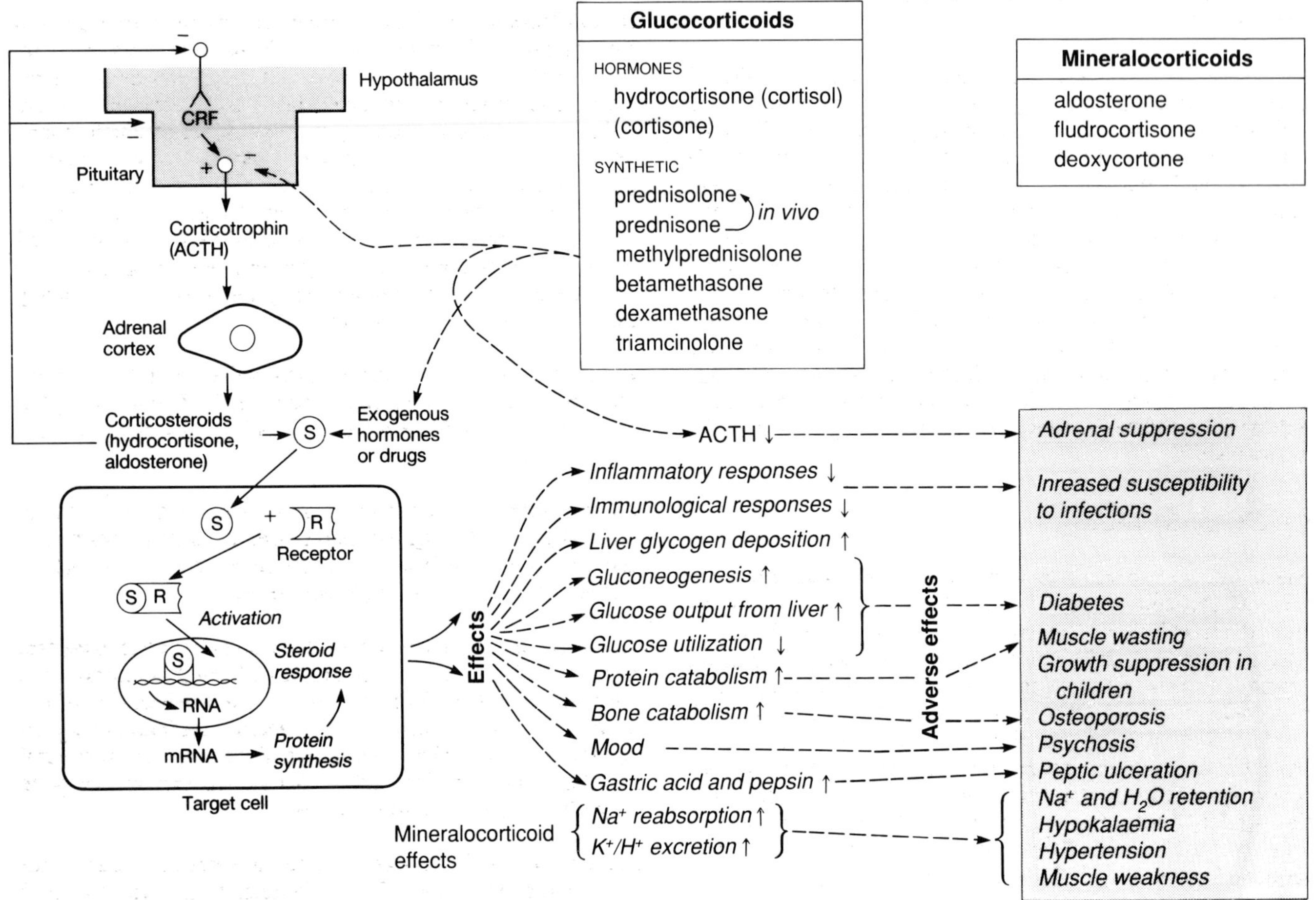

The adrenal cortex releases several steroid hormones into the circulation. They are divided by their actions into two classes. **Mineralocorticoids**, mainly aldosterone in humans, have salt-retaining activity and are synthesized in the cells of the zona glomerulosa. **Glucocorticoids**, mainly cortisol (hydrocortisone) in humans, affect carbohydrate and protein metabolism, but also have significant mineralocorticoid activity. They are synthesized in the cells of the zona fasciculata and zona reticularis.

The release of cortisol is controlled by a negative-feedback mechanism involving the hypothalamus and anterior pituitary (upper figure, ▢). Low plasma cortisol levels result in the release of corticotrophin (ACTH), which stimulates cortisol synthesis and release, probably by a mechanism involving adenylyl cyclase. Aldosterone release is affected by ACTH but other factors (e.g. renin–angiotensin system, plasma potassium) are more important.

The steroids are examples of **gene-active** hormones. These produce their effects on cells (lower figure) by promoting the synthesis of specific messenger RNA (mRNA) and so stimulate the synthesis of proteins which then produce the characteristic actions of the hormones (middle bottom).

The steroid **hormones** (*hydrocortisone* or *cortisone*) are given with a synthetic mineralocorticoid, usually **fludrocortisone** (top right), for replacement therapy in patients with adrenal insufficiency (e.g. in Addison's disease). For most therapeutic uses, synthetic glucocorticoids (top middle) have replaced the natural hormones, mainly because they have little or no salt-retaining activity.

Glucocorticoids (often *prednisolone*) are used to suppress inflammation, allergy and immune responses. Anti-inflammatory therapy is used in many diseases (e.g. rheumatoid arthritis, ulcerative colitis, bronchial asthma, severe inflammatory conditions of the eye and skin). Suppression of the immune system is of value in preventing rejection following tissue transplantation. Steroids are also used to suppress lymphopoiesis in patients with certain leukaemias and lymphomas.

Steroids can produce striking improvement in certain diseases, but high doses and prolonged use may cause **severe adverse effects** (right, ▢). These are usually predictable from the known actions of the drugs.

CRF (corticotrophin releasing factor) is a 41 amino acid polypeptide (CRF-41) whose action is enhanced by arginine vasopressin (AVP). They are produced in the hypothalamus and reach the adenohypophysis in the hypothalamo–hypophysial portal system, where they stimulate the release of corticotrophin.

Corticotrophin (adrenocorticotrophic hormone, ACTH) is processed from a large molecular weight precursor, pro-opiomelanocortin (POMC) present in corticotroph cells of the adenohypophysis and its main action is to stimulate the synthesis and release of *cortisol* (hydrocortisone). POMC also contains the sequence for *β-lipotropin* (β-LPH) which is concomitantly released into the blood. β-LPH has no known physiological effect, but it contains the sequence of *β-endorphin* and this is found in the circulation, but its relevance is debatable. However, POMC is present in the brain and there is little doubt that this is an important source for the *endorphins* within the nervous system. Corticotrophin is also believed to sensitize the zona glomerulosa to other stimuli, which cause aldosterone release (i.e. low plasma Na^+, high plasma K^+, angiotensin II).

CORTICOSTEROIDS

Mechanisms of action. The steroid hormones (glucocorticoids, mineralocorticoids and sex steroids) and synthetic corticosteroids all act by a similar general mechanism. The hormone or drug enters the cell and binds reversibly to a specific *cytoplasmic receptor.* The steroid–receptor complex then undergoes a reaction ('activation') which enables it to enter the nucleus where it binds to sites on the chromatin. The steroid–receptor complex regulates transcription of specific gene sequences into RNA molecules which are then processed to mRNAs. These leave the nucleus and bind to ribosomes, where their nucleotide sequences are translated into the corresponding amino acid sequences of proteins and specific enzymes.

GLUCOCORTICOIDS

Hydrocortisone is used: (1) orally for replacement therapy; (2) intravenously in shock and status asthmaticus; and (3) topically (e.g. ointments in eczema, enemas in ulcerative colitis).

Prednisolone is the most widely used drug given orally in inflammatory and allergic diseases.

Betamethasone and dexamethasone are very potent and have no salt-retaining actions. This makes them especially useful for high-dose therapy in conditions such as cerebral oedema where water retention would be a disadvantage.

Beclomethasone is the dipropionate ester of betamethasone. It passes membranes poorly and is more active topically than when given orally. It is used in asthma (as an aerosol) and topically in severe eczema to provide a local anti-inflammatory action with minimal systemic effects.

Triamcinolone is used in severe asthma and by intra-articular injection for local inflammation of joints.

Effects. *Glucocorticoids* influence most cells in the body.

Metabolic effects. Glucocorticoids stimulate gluconeogenesis (by increasing enzyme activity) and increase amino acid uptake by the liver and kidney. Blood glucose levels are increased, causing insulin release.

Anti-inflammatory effects. Corticosteroids have profound anti-inflammatory effects and are widely used for this purpose. Inflammation is probably suppressed by several mechanisms. Circulating immunocompetent cells and macrophages are reduced and the formation of pro-inflammatory mediators such as prostaglandins, leukotrienes and platelet activating factor (PAF) are inhibited. Steroids produce these latter effects by stimulating the synthesis in leucocytes of a protein ('lipocortin') that inhibits phospholipase A_2. This enzyme, located in the cell membrane, is activated in damaged cells and is responsible for the formation of arachidonic acid, the precursor of many inflammatory mediators (Chapter 30).

Immunosuppressive effects. Glucocorticoids inhibit complement, migration inhibition factor (MIF), T and B lymphocyte function and decrease circulating macrophages and lymphocytes.

Adverse effects. Glucocorticoids produce many adverse effects, especially with the high doses required for anti-inflammatory activity. (Similar effects are produced by the excess corticosteroids secreted in Cushing's syndrome.)

Metabolic effects. High doses quickly cause a rounded, plethoric face (moon face) and fat is redistributed from the extremities to the trunk and face. Purple striae and a tendency to bruise develop. Disturbed carbohydrate metabolism leads to hyperglycaemia and occasionally diabetes. Protein loss from skeletal muscles causes wasting and weakness. An increase in bone catabolism may cause osteoporosis.

Fluid retention, hypokalaemia and hypertension may occur with compounds that have significant mineralocorticoid activity. Thus, hydrocortisone (and cortisone) are generally used only for replacement therapy in adrenal insufficiency.

Adrenal suppression. Steroid therapy suppresses corticotrophin secretion and this eventually leads to adrenal atrophy. It may take 6–12 months for normal adrenal function to recover once therapy is stopped. Since the patient's response to stress is suppressed, additional steroid must be administered in times of severe stress (e.g. surgery, infection). Steroid therapy must be withdrawn very gradually, because abrupt withdrawal causes adrenal insufficiency.

Infections. There is increased susceptibility to infections, which may progress unrecognized because the natural indicators of infection are inhibited.

Other complications include psychosis, cataracts, glaucoma, peptic ulceration and the reactivation of nascent infections (e.g. tuberculosis).

MINERALOCORTICOIDS

Fludrocortisone or deoxycortone are given with hydrocortisone in adrenal insufficiency (e.g. Addison's disease or following adrenalectomy) because the latter drug does not possess sufficient salt-retaining activity.

32 Sex hormones and drugs

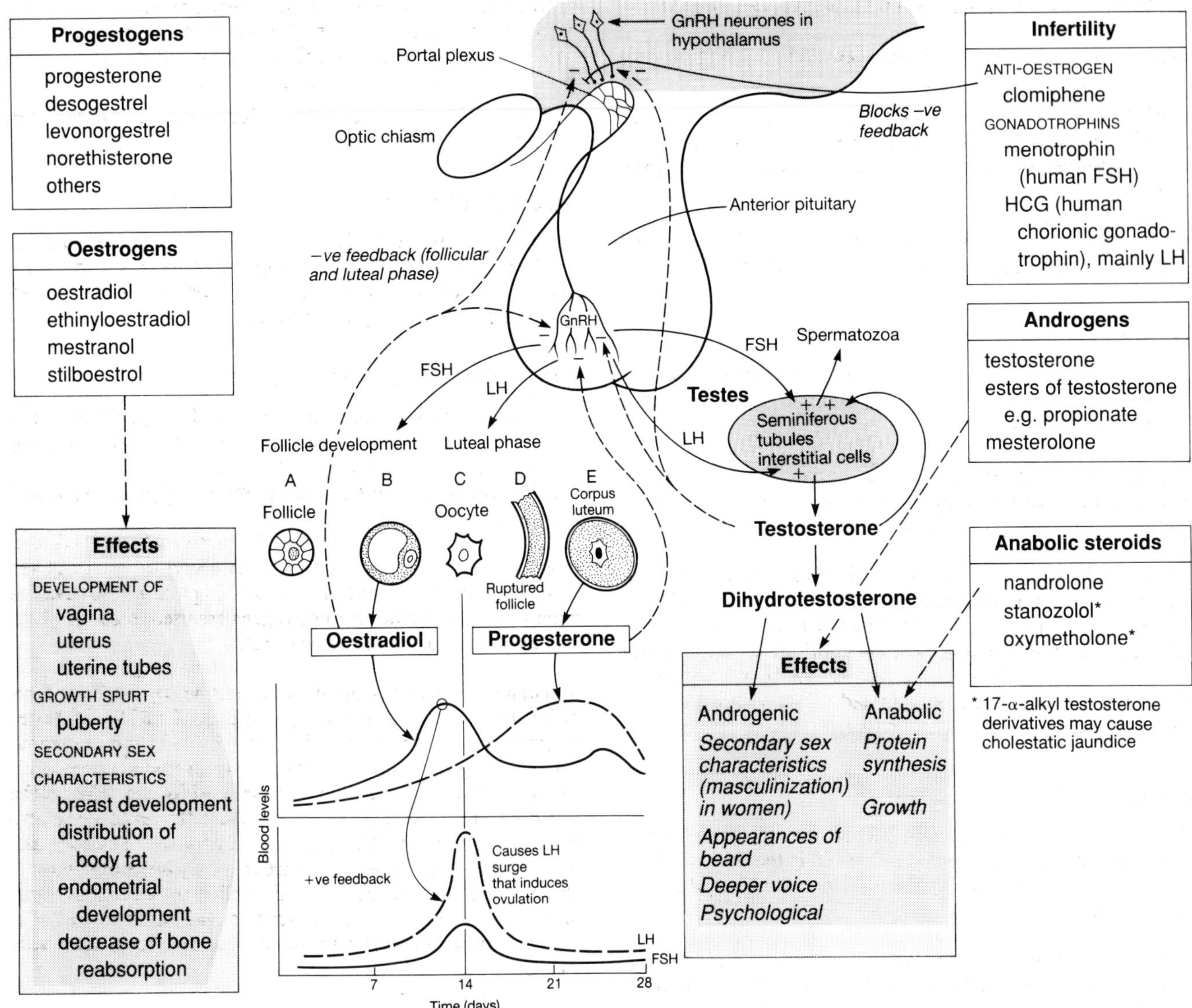

The ovaries and testes, in addition to producing gametes, also secrete hormones (mainly **oestrogens** and **androgens**, respectively). The secretion of oestrogens (mainly oestradiol) and androgens (mainly testosterone) requires **gonadotrophins** (luteinizing and follicle stimulating hormones, LH and FSH) which are hormones released from the anterior pituitary (middle top). The release of LH and FSH are in turn controlled by the hypothalamus (top, ▢), which releases pulses of gonadotrophin-releasing hormone (GnRH).

In the **testes** (right, ⬭), spermatozoa are produced in the seminiferous tubules by a process requiring both FSH and *testosterone*, the latter hormone being synthesized in the interstitial cells in response to LH. Testosterone causes the changes that occur in the normal male at puberty (bottom right, shaded). **Androgens** (middle right) are used mainly for replacement therapy in castrated males or in males who are hypogonadal due to either pituitary or testicular disease. *Testosterone* is rapidly inactivated by the liver following oral administration, but synthetic androgens (e.g. mesterolone) are active orally. **Anabolic steroids** (bottom right) have relatively little androgenic activity and are used to try and increase protein synthesis after major surgery and in chronic debilitating disease. The main adverse effects of androgens, and, to a lesser extent, the anabolic steroids, is masculinization in women and perpubertal children and the suppression of FSH and LH.

In the **ovary**, FSH (and LH) stimulate follicular development (top left A–B) and *oestradiol* synthesis by the granulosa cells of the follicle. In the early follicular phase, the low oestradiol level in the blood (middle left) exerts a negative feedback effect on FSH, ensuring that only the dominant follicle ripens. Midway through the cycle, oestradiol levels are high and this has a positive feedback effect on LH secretion, leading to the 'LH surge' (bottom left) which causes ovulation. These feedback effects of oestradiol are exerted on the hypothalamus (changing the amount of GnRH secreted) and the pituitary gland (altering its response to GnRH). The ruptured follicle (D) develops into the corpus luteum (E), which secretes oestrogen and progesterone (middle left) until the end of the cycle. During the follicular phase of the cycle, oestrogen stimulates endometrial proliferation. In the luteal phase, increased progesterone release stimulates the maturation and glandular development of the endometrium, which is then shed in the process of menstruation.

Oestrogens (middle left) have many effects (bottom left, shaded). They are used for replacement therapy in primary hypogonadism and in postmenopausal women to prevent hot flushes, atrophic vaginitis and osteoporosis. They are also used in a number of menstrual disorders (e.g. spasmodic dysmenorrhoea), and in combination with progestogens, as contraceptives. Progestogens (top left) are used mainly for hormonal contraception. Sex hormones and antagonists are used in the treatment of certain cancers (Chapter 40).

GnRH (gonadotrophin-releasing hormone) is a decapeptide that stimulates FSH and LH release from the anterior pituitary gland. Pulsatile infusions of GnRH are used to treat hypothalamic hypogonadism.

LH and **FSH** are glycoprotein hormones produced by the anterior pituitary. They regulate gonadal function.

INFERTILITY

In anovulatory women, infertility may be overcome providing the ovary is capable of producing a mature ova and the appropriate steroids.

Clomiphene and tamoxifen are anti-oestrogens. They work by inhibiting the feedback inhibition of oestrogens in the hypothalamus and so increase FSH and LH release.

Gonadotrophins are used in women lacking appropriate pituitary function or not responding to clomiphene therapy. Treatment starts with daily injections of menotrophin (mainly FSH) followed by one or two large doses of chorionic gonadotrophin (mainly LH). Multiple births occur in 20–30% of pregnancies after treatment. In men, both gonadotrophins are given to stimulate spermatogenesis and androgen release.

TESTOSTERONE

The most important androgen in humans is testosterone. About 2% of testosterone in the plasma is free and in the skin, prostate, seminal vesicles and epididymis it is converted to dihydrotestosterone.

Effects. At puberty, androgens cause development of the secondary sexual characteristics in the male. In the adult male, large doses suppress the release of gonadotrophins and cause some atrophy of the interstitial tissue and tubules of the testes. *Testosterone enanthate* given by weekly injections has recently been shown to provide highly effective, reversible contraception in most men by inducing azoospermia, but potential long-term effects might include prostate and cardiovascular disease. In women, androgens cause changes, many of which are similar to those seen in the prepubertal male.

OESTROGENS

Oestradiol is the main oestrogen released by the human ovary. Synthetic oestrogens are more effective following oral administration.

Adverse effects (see oral contraceptives). The continuous administration of oestrogens for prolonged periods can cause abnormal endometrial hyperplasia, abnormal bleeding patterns, and is associated with an increased incidence of endometrial carcinoma. When a progestogen is given with the oestrogen, there is a decreased incidence of ovarian and endometrial cancers.

PROGESTOGENS

Progestogens are used for hormonal contraception and for producing long-term ovarian suppression for other purposes (e.g. dysmenorrhoea, endometriosis, hirsutism and bleeding disorders) when oestrogens are contraindicated.

ORAL CONTRACEPTIVES

Combination pills contain oestrogen and progestogen. They are taken for 20–21 days and discontinued for the following 6–7 days to allow menstruation to occur.

Mini-progestogen pills contain a low dose of progestogen and are taken continuously.

Only two oestrogens are used: mestranol and ethinyloestradiol. Both compounds have an acetylene group at the 17-α position, which appears to slow hepatic metabolism. A wide variety of synthetic progestogens are used, most of which are derivatives of 19-nortestosterone.

Mechanism of action. Combination pills act by feedback inhibition on the hypothalamus to suppress GnRH and hence plasma gonadotrophin secretion, thereby blocking ovulation. These drugs also produce an endometrium that is unreceptive to implantation, alter Fallopian tube motility, and change the composition of cervical mucus. These latter effects are also produced by mini-progestogen pills and appear to be the basis of their contraceptive actions, since they only block ovulation in about 25% of women. Menstruation often ceases initially with mini-progestogens, but usually returns with prolonged administration. However, the length and duration of bleeding are very variable.

Adverse effects. *Non-life threatening* side-effects that occur with both combination pills and mini-progestogens include breakthrough bleeding, weight gain, changes in libido, breast soreness, headache and nausea. Combination pills may also cause hirsutism, vaginal yeast infections and depression. About 20–30% of women will experience some of these effects and 10–15% will stop taking the pill because of them. The overall incidence of side-effects is lower with mini-progestogens, but breakthrough bleeding and irregular menses are major complaints with these drugs.

Serious side-effects are rare. They include cholestatic jaundice and a six- to eight-fold greater incidence of thromboembolic disease, for which the oestrogen is apparently responsible.

'Abortion pill'. Progesterone supports endometrial nidation of the fertilized ovum and the progesterone antagonist, *mifepristone*, has been found to be highly effective in terminating early pregnancy when used with a prostaglandin cervical ripening agent (usually gemeprost or sulprostone pessaries). The main adverse effects are pain and bleeding, which may be severe.

33 Thyroid and antithyroid drugs

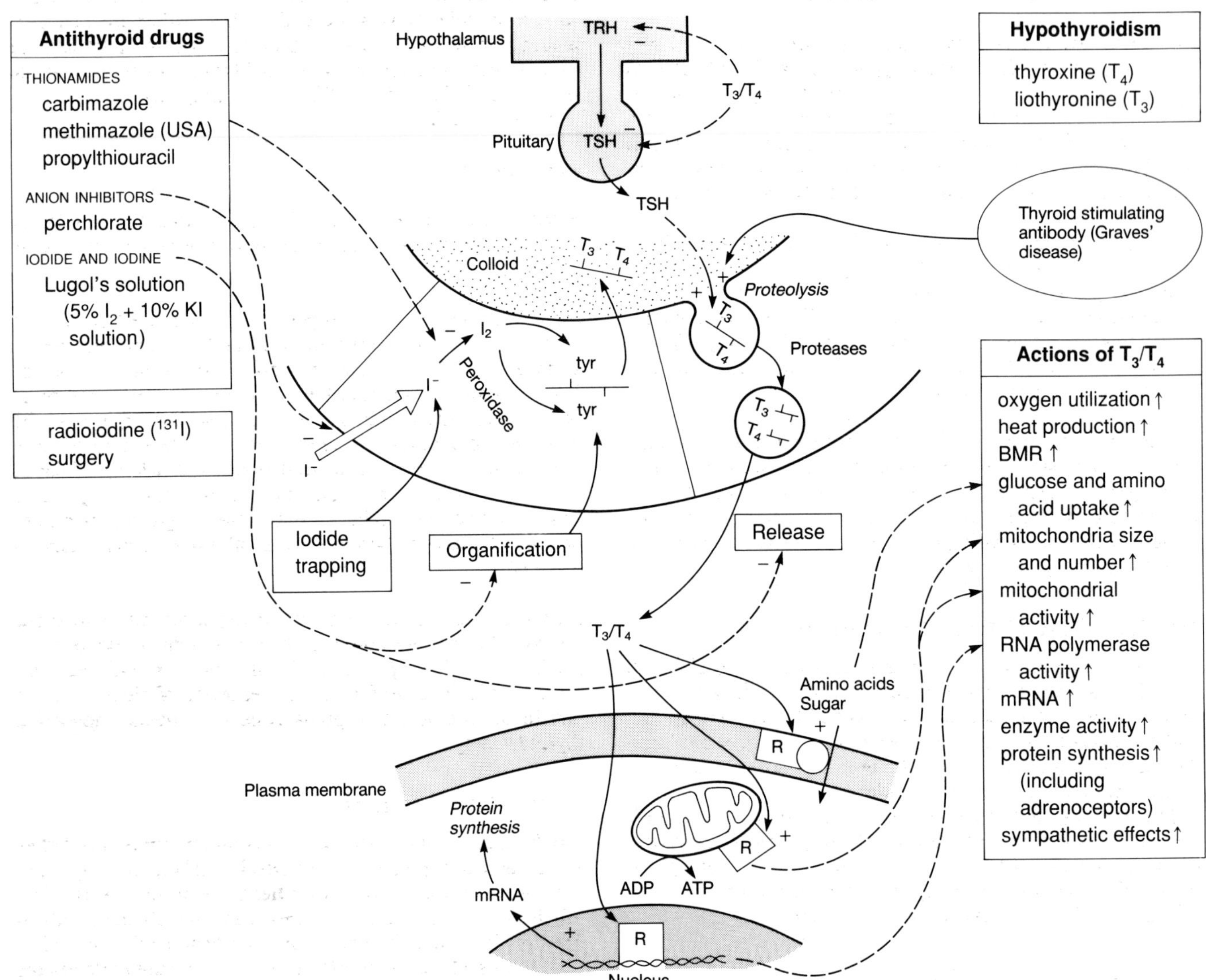

The thyroid gland secretes two iodinated hormones called **triiodothyronine (T_3)** and **thyroxine** (tetraiodothyronine, **T_4**) which are responsible for the optimal growth, development, function and maintenance of body tissues. Another hormone, **calcitonin**, is produced by the parafollicular cells and is involved in the regulation of calcium metabolism.

The synthesis of T_3 and T_4 requires **iodine**, which is normally ingested (as iodide) in the diet. An active, *thyrotrophin-dependent* pump (⇨) concentrates the **iodide** in the follicular cells (centre figure) where it is rapidly oxidized by a peroxidase catalysed reaction to the more reactive **iodine**. The iodine reacts with tyrosine residues present in thyroglobulin ('organification') and units of T_3 and T_4 are formed. The thyroglobulin containing these iodothyronines is then secreted into the follicles and stored as colloid (▒).

The release of T_3 and T_4 is controlled by a negative feedback system (top figure). When the circulating levels of T_3 and T_4 fall, **thyrotrophin (TSH)** is released from the anterior pituitary gland and stimulates the transport of colloid into the follicular cells. Then, the colloid droplets fuse with lysosomes, and protease enzymes degrade the thyroglobulin, releasing T_3 and T_4 into the circulation. Both thyroid hormones act on receptors (R) in the plasma membrane and on intracellular receptors (bottom figure) to produce a variety of actions (right).

Thyroid hyperfunction and hypofunction occur in about 2% of the population and together with diabetes mellitus (2–3% of the population) are the most common endocrine disorders. In **Graves' disease**, hyperthyroidism is produced by an antibody that causes prolonged activation of the TSH receptors and results in excessive secretion of T_3 and T_4. Thyroid activity can be reduced with drugs that reduce hormone synthesis (left), or by the destruction of the gland with radiation (using ^{131}I) or surgery. Hyperthyroidism often causes increased sympathetic effects which can be blocked with β-adrenoceptor antagonists (e.g. propranolol). Graves' disease is often associated with ophthalmopathy which is often difficult to control and may be a distinct organ-specific autoimmune disease.

Primary hypothyroidism (**myxoedema**) probably results in most cases from a cell-mediated immune response directed against the thyroid follicular cells. Thyroxine is the drug of choice for replacement therapy (top right).

TRH. Thyrotrophin-releasing hormone is a tripeptide synthesized in the hypothalamus and transported in the capillaries of the pituitary portal venous system to the pituitary gland where it stimulates TSH synthesis and release.

TSH. Thyrotrophin is a glycoprotein hormone which is released from the pituitary gland (adenohypophysis) and stimulates the synthesis and release of hormones from the thyroid gland. In hypothyroidism or (rarely) iodine deficiency, abnormally high levels of TSH result in the enlargement of the thyroid gland (goitre). *Goitrogens* are chemicals that suppress thyroid hormone function, resulting in elevated TSH and goitre.

T_3 and T_4. Triiodothyronine and thyroxine (tetraiodothyronine) enter the circulation, where they are transported largely bound to plasma proteins (99.5% and 99.95%, respectively). The thyroid only contributes about 20% of the unbound circulating T_3, the remainder being produced by the *peripheral conversion* of T_4 to T_3. T_4 may also be deiodinated to inactive reverse T_3 according to the demands of the tissues.

Actions. The mechanisms of action of the thyroid hormones are not fully understood, but are thought to involve high-affinity binding sites (receptors) in the *plasma membrane*, *mitochondria* and *nucleus*. These receptor–hormone interactions result in a variety of effects, including increased protein synthesis and an increase in energy metabolism.

HYPERTHYROIDISM (*thyrotoxicosis*)

The basal metabolic rate is increased, causing heat intolerance, arrhythmias and increased appetite. The skin is warm and moist. There is increased nervousness and hyperkinesia. Sympathetic overactivity causes tachycardia, sweating and tremor. Angina and high-output heart failure may occur. The upper eyelids are retracted, causing a wide stare.

Traditionally, young patients have been treated with antithyroid drugs and, if the condition relapses, subtotal thyroidectomy. Over about 40 years of age, patients have been given radioiodine therapy. Nowadays young patients may be given ^{131}I and carbimazole may be given long term.

ANTITHYROID DRUGS

Thionamides possess a thiocarbamide group (S = C – N) which is essential for their activity. They prevent the synthesis of thyroid hormones by competitively inhibiting the peroxidase catalysed reactions necessary for iodine organification. They also block the coupling of the iodotyrosine, especially diiodothyronine formation. Thionamides may be immunosuppressive, but this is controversial. All the antithyroid drugs are administered orally and are accumulated in the thyroid gland. Their onset of action is delayed until the preformed hormones are depleted, a process that may take 3–4 weeks.

Carbimazole is rapidly converted to methimazole *in vivo*. The aim is to render the patient euthyroid and then to give a reduced dose for maintenance. It is often possible to cease treatment after 1 or 2 years. Side-effects include rashes and, rarely, agranulocytosis.

Propylthiouracil is usually reserved for patients intolerant to carbimazole. It is associated with a higher incidence of agranulocyosis (0.4%) than carbimazole (0.1%). In addition to inhibiting hormone synthesis, propylthiouracil also inhibits the peripheral de-iodination of T_4 and perhaps has an immunosuppressive action.

Anion inhibitors

Potassium perchlorate competitively inhibits the uptake of iodine by the thyroid. It is not used now, as it may cause aplastic anaemia.

Iodine. Iodides have several poorly understood actions on the thyroid. They inhibit organification and hormone release. In addition, iodide decreases the size and vascularity of the hyperplastic gland, effects which are useful in the preparation of patients for thyroidectomy. In 'pharmacological' doses, the main effect of iodides is to inhibit hormone release and, because thyrotoxic symptoms are reduced relatively quickly (2–7 days), iodine is valuable in the treatment of thyroid storm (thyrotoxic crisis). Iodine cannot be used for the long-term treatment of hyperthyroidism because its antithyroid action tends to diminish.

Propranolol or atenolol can reduce the heart rate and other sympathetic manifestations of hyperthyroidism and provide partial relief of symptoms until full control is achieved with carbimazole. It is useful in the treatment of thyroid storm and in the pre-operative preparation of patients undergoing thyroidectomy.

HYPOTHYROIDISM

Tiredness and lethargy are the most common symptoms. Other effects include depression of the basal metabolic rate, appetite and cardiac output. Low-output heart failure may occur. The skin is dry. Thyroid hormone deprivation in early life results in irreversible mental retardation and dwarfism (cretinism) and to prevent this, all newborn infants are screened and replacement therapy given from birth.

REPLACEMENT THERAPY

Thyroxine administered orally is the treatment of choice. Synthetic T_4 is the sodium salt of L-thyroxine. Its effects are delayed until the plasma protein and tissue binding sites are occupied. Treatment can be assessed by monitoring plasma TSH levels, which fall to normal when the optimum dose is achieved.

Liothyronine is the sodium salt of T_3 and because it is less protein bound, it acts more quickly than T_4. The main use of T_3 is in hypothyroid coma, when it is given (together with hydrocortisone) by intravenous injection.

34 Antidiabetic agents

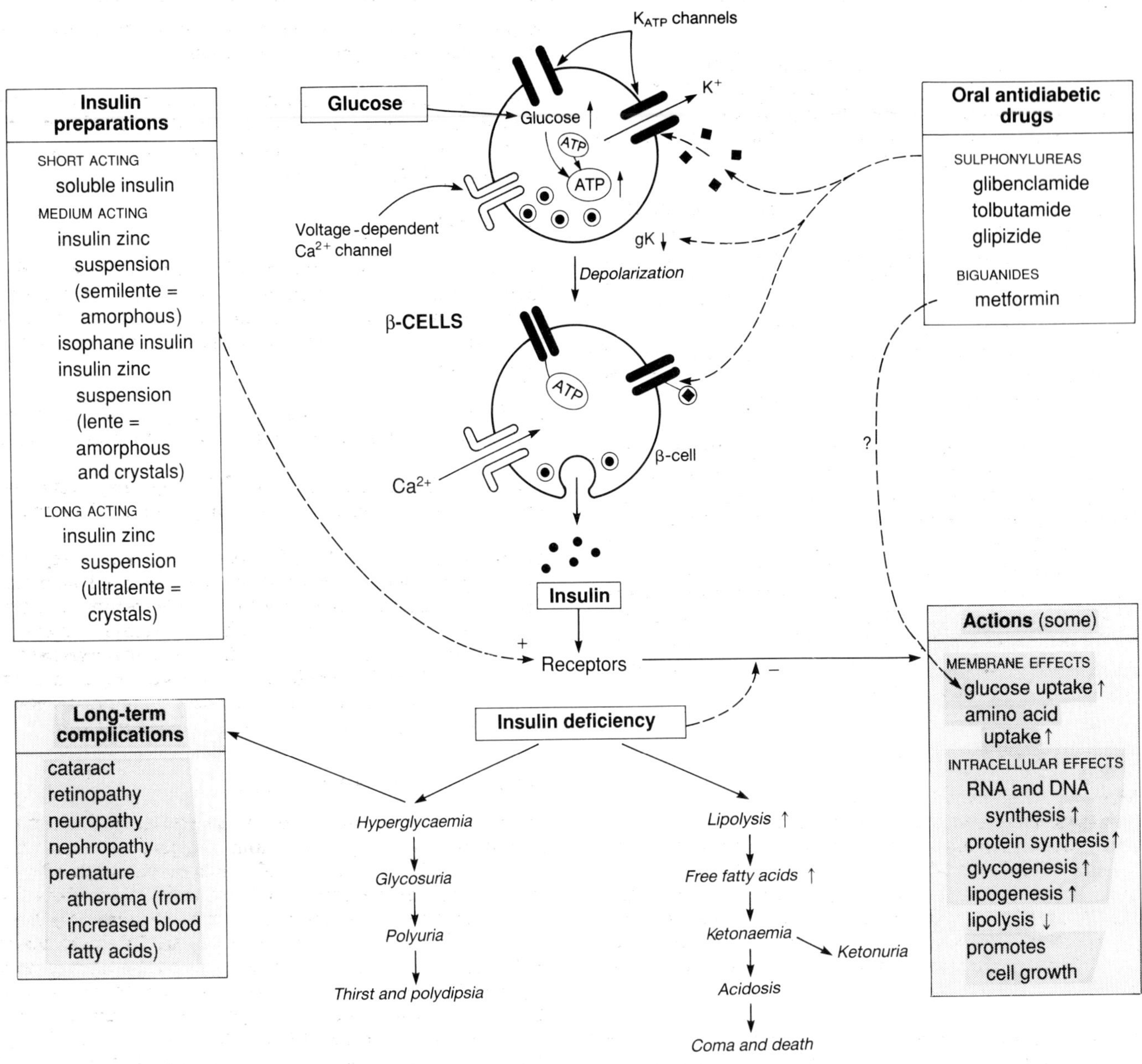

Insulin is a hormone secreted by the β-cells of the islets of Langerhans in the pancreas (top). Various stimuli **release** insulin (●) from storage granules (⦿) in the β-cells, but the most potent stimulus is a rise in plasma glucose (hyperglycaemia). Insulin binds to specific **receptors** in the cell membranes, initiating a number of actions (bottom right, shaded) including an increase of glucose uptake by muscle, liver and adipose tissue.

In **diabetes mellitus** there is a relative or total absence of insulin, which causes reduced glucose uptake by insulin-sensitive tissues and has serious consequences (middle bottom). Lipolysis and muscle proteolysis result in weight loss and weakness. The blood levels of free fatty acids and glycerol rise. An excess of acetyl-CoA is produced in the liver and converted to *acetoacetic acid*, which is then either reduced to *β-hydroxybutyric* acid or decarboxylated to *acetone*. These 'ketone bodies' accumulate in the blood, causing an acidosis (ketoacidosis). About 25% of diabetics have a severe deficiency of insulin. This **Type I** or **insulin-dependent diabetes** is associated with HLA antigens and immunological selective β-cell destruction. In these patients, *ketosis* is common and insulin is required. Various **insulin preparations** (top left) and **regimens** are used. There is evidence that metabolic control early in the course of the disease may prevent or delay the onset of diabetic complications (bottom left, shaded). In **Type II** or **non-insulin dependent diabetes** the aetiology is unknown, but a strong genetic component is present. There is a resistance to circulating insulin, which does, however, protect the patient from ketosis. There is a reduction in the number of insulin receptors which is often associated with obesity. Loss of weight (diet and exercise) reduces insulin 'resistance' and controls about one-third of Type II diabetics. Another one-third of Type II diabetics are controlled by diet together with **oral antidiabetic drugs** (top right). The **sulphonylureas (■)** close K_{ATP} channels (middle) causing depolarization of the β-cells and increased insulin release. Type II diabetics not controlled by diet and oral antidiabetic drugs require insulin injections. These tend to be the thinner patients who lack the first phase insulin response.

INSULIN

Insulin is a protein containing 51 amino acids arranged in two chains (A and B) linked by disulphide bridges. A precursor, called pro-insulin is hydrolysed inside storage granules to form insulin and a residual C-peptide. The granules store insulin as crystals, containing zinc and insulin.

Release. Glucose is the most potent stimulus for insulin release from islet β-cells. There is a continuous basal secretion with surges at feeding times. The β-cells possess K^+ channels that are regulated by intracellular ATP (K_{ATP} channels). When the blood glucose increases, more glucose enters the β-cells and its metabolism results in an increase in intracellular ATP which closes the K_{ATP} channels. The resulting depolarization of the β-cell initiates an influx of Ca^{2+} ions through voltage-sensitive Ca^{2+} channels, which triggers insulin release.

Insulin receptors are membrane-spanning glycoproteins consisting of two α-subunits and two β-subunits linked covalently by disulphide bonds. After insulin binds to the α-subunit, the insulin receptor complex enters the cell, where it is eventually destroyed by lysosomal enzymes. The internalization of the insulin receptor complex may underlie the *downregulation* of receptors that is produced by high levels of insulin (e.g. in obese subjects). The mechanisms linking insulin-receptor activation to the actions of insulin are not understood, but a tyrosine kinase activity of the β-subunit and its autophosphorylation seem essential for insulin action.

INSULIN PREPARATIONS

Most diabetics in the United Kingdom are now treated with human insulin prepared by recombinant DNA technology, although some remain on insulin prepared from porcine or beef pancreas. Insulin is administered by subcutaneous injection and its rate of *absorption* can be prolonged by *increasing the particle size* (i.e. crystals slower than amorphous) or by *complexing the insulin with zinc or protamine.* Insulin preparations are classified traditionally into *short, intermediate,* and *long acting.*

Short-acting preparations. *Soluble insulin* is a simple solution of insulin. (Onset 30 minutes, peak activity 1–3 hours, duration 7 hours). It can be administered intravenously in hyperglycaemic emergencies.

Medium-acting preparations have a duration of action between 14 and 22 hours. *Semilente* is a suspension of amorphous insulin zinc. *Lente* is a mixture of amorphous insulin zinc (30%) and insulin zinc crystals (70%), the latter prolonging the duration of this preparation.

Isophane insulin (NPH) is a complex of protamine and insulin. The mixture is such that no free binding sites remain on the protamine. After injection, proteolytic enzymes degrade the protamine and the insulin is absorbed. The duration of NPH is similar to that of *lente* (about 20 hours).

Biphasic fixed mixtures contain various proportions of soluble and isophane insulin (e.g. 30% soluble and 70% isophane). The soluble component gives a rapid onset and the isophane insulin prolongs the action.

Long-acting preparations. *Ultralente* is a suspension of poorly soluble insulin zinc crystals that has a duration of 36 hours. The long duration of *ultralente* can lead to insulin accumulation and dangerous hypoglycaemia.

Adverse effects

Hypoglycaemia due to insulin overdose or inadequate calorific intake is the most common and most serious complication of insulin treatment. If severe, coma and death will occur if the patient is not treated with glucose (intravenously if unconscious).

Insulin antibodies. All insulins are immunogenic to some extent (bovine most) but immunological resistance to insulin is rare.

Local allergic reactions at the injection site may occur and *lipohypertrophy* is common with all preparations of insulin.

Insulin regimens. Most Type I diabetic patients use a regimen involving a combination of short- and intermediate-acting insulin injected subcutaneously twice daily, before breakfast and before the evening meal. More demanding, intensive control regimens, designed to produce near normoglycaemia may reduce diabetic complications (one such regimen is an injection of ultralente insulin to provide a background level of insulin and soluble insulin three times a day before meals).

ORAL ANTIDIABETIC DRUGS

Sulphonylureas are indicated in patients (especially those near their ideal weight) in whom diet fails to control the hyperglycaemia, but in about 30% control is not achieved with these drugs. These agents stimulate insulin release from the pancreatic islets and so the patient must have *partially functional β-cells* for these drugs to be of use. **Glibenclamide** is widely used and is sometimes effective when tolbutamide fails. If glibenclamide fails, other drugs are unlikely to be effective. **Tolbutamide** is less potent than glibenclamide but its short duration of action makes it the preferred drug in the elderly. Tobutamide (and glipizide) are metabolized in the liver and therefore may be especially useful in renal failure.

Adverse effects. Gastrointestinal disturbances and rashes occur, but are rare. Hypoglycaemia and hypoglycaemic coma may be induced by longer-acting drugs, *especially in elderly patients.* Sulphonylureas are contraindicated in severe (especially ketotic) hyperglycaemia, surgery and major illness, when insulin should be given.

Biguanides. *Metformin* acts peripherally to increase glucose uptake by an unknown mechanism. As it does not increase insulin release, it rarely causes hypoglycaemia. Metformin may act synergistically with sulphonylureas and therefore may avoid the need for insulin injections. Adverse effects include nausea, vomiting, diarrhoea, malaise and, very occasionally, fatal lactic acidosis.

35 Antimicrobial drugs that inhibit nucleic acid synthesis: sulphonamides, trimethoprim and quinolones

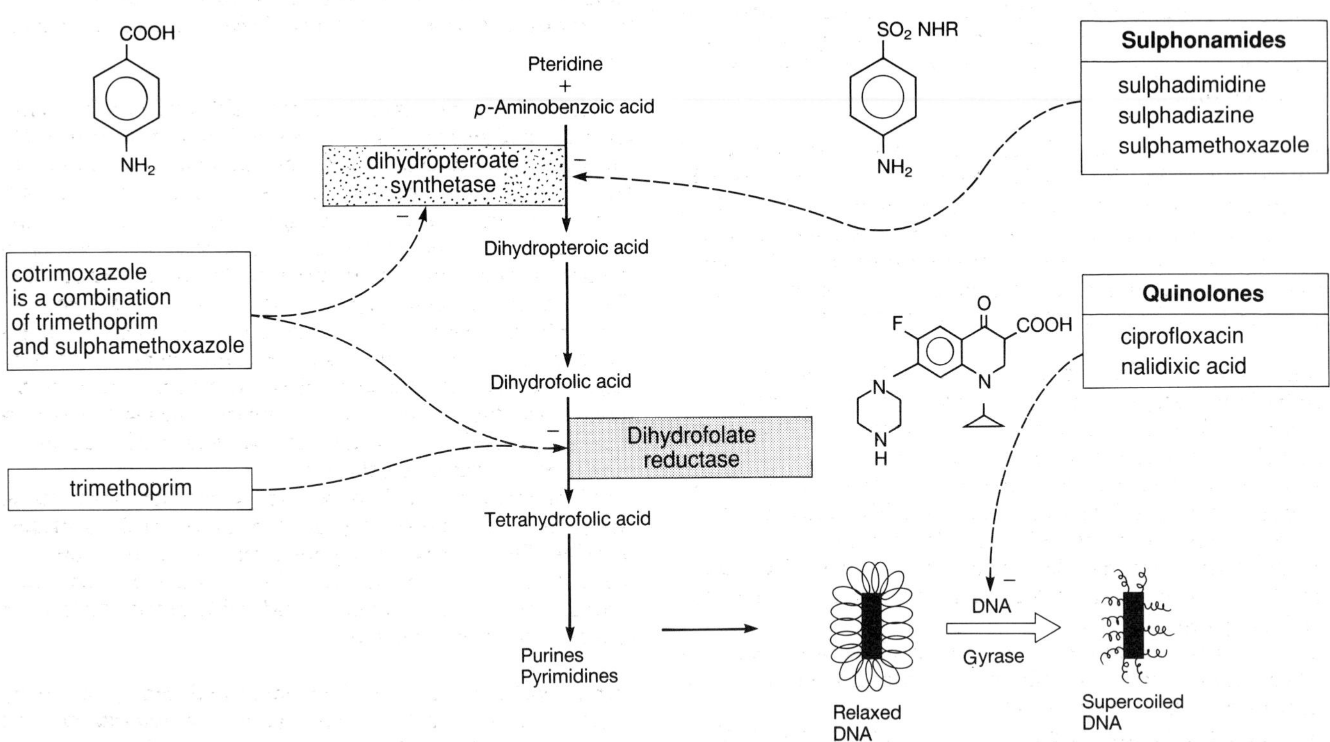

The sulphonamides were the first drugs found to be effective in the treatment of systemic infections. However, they are now of little importance because of the development of more effective agents which are less toxic. Also, many organisms have developed **resistance** to sulphonamides. Their principal use alone is in the treatment of urinary tract infections caused by sensitive Gram-positive or Gram-negative organisms.*

There are many sulphonamides and a few examples are given together with their general structure (top right). They are structural analogues of *p*-aminobenzoic acid (top left) which is essential for folic acid synthesis in bacteria. The **selective toxicity** of the sulphonamides depends on the fact that mammalian cells take up folate supplied in the diet, but susceptible bacteria lack this ability and must synthesize folate. Sulphonamides competitively inhibit the enzyme dihydropteroate synthetase (▨), and prevent the production of folate required for the synthesis of DNA. The sulphonamides are **bacteriostatic** agents. Their most important side-effects are rashes (common), renal failure and various blood dyscrasias.

Trimethoprim (bottom left) acts on the same metabolic pathway as sulphonamides, but is an inhibitor of dihydrofolate reductase (▨). It is selectively toxic because its affinity for the bacterial enzyme is 50 000 times greater than its affinity for the human enzyme. Trimethoprim is increasingly used alone, but a combination of trimethoprim and sulphamethoxazole (**cotrimoxazole**) (left) may produce a synergistic action and increased activity against certain bacteria. Trimethoprim and cotrimoxazole are used mainly in the treatment of urinary tract and respiratory infections.

The **4-quinolones** (middle right) inhibit DNA gyrase, an enzyme that compresses bacterial DNA into supercoils (⇨). Inhibition of DNA gyrase is believed to lead to unwinding of the supercoils and, ultimately, cell death. **Ciprofloxacin** is a recently introduced broad-spectrum antibacterial agent that is increasingly used. Important properties of the quinolones are their good penetration into tissues and cells (cf. penicillins) and their effectiveness when given orally.

* Bacteria are classified by their shape (cocci are spherical, bacilli are rod-shaped) and many by whether (Gram-positive) or not (Gram-negative) they remain stained with methyl violet after washing with acetone. The retention or not of methyl violet reflects important differences in the bacterial cell walls.

Selective toxicity. The use of chemicals to try and eradicate parasites, bacteria, viruses or cancer cells in the body is called chemotherapy. It depends on the drugs being selectively toxic, i.e. toxic to the cells of the parasite, but not (too) toxic to the human host. Bacteria have many biochemical differences from human cells, and some antibacterial drugs are strikingly non-toxic to humans. On the other hand, because cancer cells are so similar to normal cells, most anticancer drugs show little selective toxicity and therefore produce serious adverse effects (Chapter 40).

Bacteriostatic agents inhibit bacterial growth whilst **bactericidal agents** actually kill the organism. This distinction is not usually important clinically, as host defence mechanisms are involved in the final elimination of bacterial pathogens. An exception is the treatment of infections in immunocompromised patients (AIDS, corticosteroids, anticancer and immunosuppressant drugs), when a bactericidal agent should be used.

Resistance to antimicrobial drugs can be acquired or innate. In the latter case, an entire bacterial species may be resistant to a drug before its introduction. For example, *Pseudomonas aeruginosa* has always been resistant to flucloxacillin. More serious clinically is **acquired resistance**, where bacteria that were once sensitive to a drug become resistant. Mechanisms responsible for resistance to antimicrobial drugs include:

1 **Inactivating enzymes that destroy the drug**, e.g. β-lactamases produced by many staphylococci inactivate most penicillins and many cephalosporins.

2 **Decreased drug accumulation.** Tetracycline resistance occurs where the bacterial cell membrane becomes impermeable to the drug or there is increased efflux.

3 **Alteration of binding sites.** Aminoglycosides and erythromycin bind to bacterial ribosomes and inhibit protein synthesis. In resistant organisms, the sites of drug binding may be modified so that they no longer have affinity for the drugs.

4 **Development of alternative metabolic pathways.** Bacteria can become resistant to sulphonamides and trimethoprim because they produce modified dihydropteroate synthetase and dihydrofolate reductase enzymes, respectively, which have little or no affinity for the drugs.

Antibiotic-resistant bacterial populations can develop in several ways.

1 **Selection.** Within a population there will be some bacteria with acquired resistance. The drug then eliminates the sensitive organisms and the resistant forms proliferate.

2 **Transferred resistance.** Here, the gene that codes for the resistance mechanism is transferred from one organism to another. The antibiotic resistance genes may be carried in **plasmids**, which are small extrachromosomal circles of DNA within the bacteria. The plasmids (and therefore antibiotic resistance) can be transferred from one organism to another by *conjugation* (the formation of a tube between the organisms). Many Gram-negative and some Gram-positive bacteria can conjugate. In *transduction*, plasmid DNA is enclosed in a bacterial virus (bacteriophage) and transferred to another organism of the same species. This is a relatively ineffective method of transfer, but is clinically important in the transfer of resistance-genes between strains of staphylococci and streptococci.

SULPHONAMIDES

Sulphadimidine and **sulphadiazine** are well absorbed following oral administration. They are metabolized mainly by acetylation, the rate of which is bimodally distributed (i.e. there are 'slow' and 'fast' acetylators—see hydralazine, Chapter 15, for another example). These drugs are used for treating 'simple' urinary tract infections but many *Escherichia coli** strains are resistant.

Adverse effects. The most common side-effects are allergic reactions and include skin rashes (morbilliform or urticarial), sometimes with a fever. Much less common are more serious reactions, e.g. the Stevens–Johnson syndrome, which is a form of erythema multiforme with a high mortality rate. Sulphonamides with a low solubility such as sulphadiazine may crystallize from the urine in the kidneys (crystalluria), causing damage. This can be prevented by making the urine alkaline with sodium bicarbonate and by maintaining a high fluid intake. It is not a problem with more soluble sulphonamides, such as sulphamethoxazole. Various blood dyscrasias may occur, rarely, including agranulocytosis, aplastic anaemia and haemolytic anaemia (especially in patients with glucose-6-phosphodehydrogenase deficiency).

Sulphonamides should not be given to neonates or women in late pregnancy because they displace bilirubin from plasma proteins. The increase in unbound bilirubin may result in it being deposited in the neonatal brain, where it may cause characteristic yellow staining and widespread destructive changes known as kernicterus.

Trimethoprim is well absorbed orally and can be given by injection. It is sometimes used alone for respiratory tract infections, but it has relatively poor activity against *Streptococcus pneumoniae* and *Streptococcus pyogenes.* **Cotrimoxazole (trimethoprim** combined with **sulphamethoxazole)** is used in urinary tract infections (*E. coli*), respiratory infections (*Haemophilus influenzae* and *pneumococci*) and, in high doses, unusual infections such as toxoplasmosis and pneumocystis. The side-effects of cotrimoxazole are mainly those of the sulphonamide.

QUINOLONES

Nalidixic acid was the first 4-quinolone found to have antibacterial activity, but it does not achieve systemic antibacterial levels and has been used only for urinary tract infections. **Ciprofloxacin** has a 6-fluoro substituent which confers greatly enhanced antibacterial potency against both Gram-positive and especially Gram-negative organisms, including *E. coli*, *Pseudomonas aeruginosa*, salmonella and campylobacter. Resistance, so far, is uncommon. Ciprofloxacin is well absorbed orally and can be given intravenously. It is eliminated, largely unchanged, mainly by the kidneys. Side-effects are infrequent but include nausea, vomiting, rashes, dizziness and headache. Convulsions may occur because the quinolones are GABA antagonists.

* *E. coli* is a Gram-negative rod and is the most common cause of urinary tract infections.

36 Antimicrobial drugs that inhibit cell wall synthesis: penicillins, cephalosporins and vancomycin

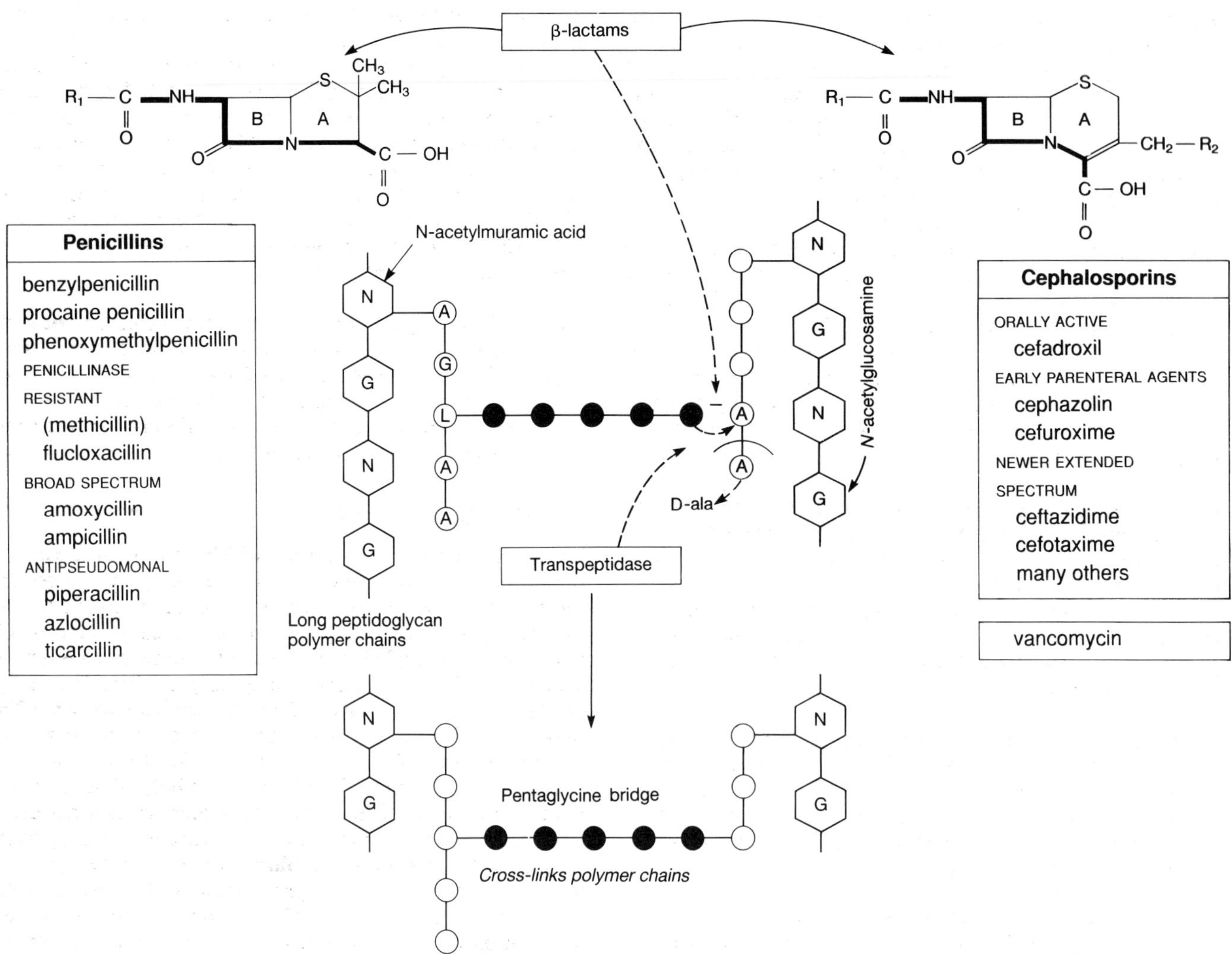

The structures of the penicillins (top left) and cephalosporins (top right) share the common feature of a β-lactam ring (B), the integrity of which is essential for antimicrobial activity. Modification of groups R_1 and R_2 have resulted in many semi-synthetic antibiotics, some of which are acid resistant (and orally active), have a wide spectrum of antimicrobial activity, or are resistant to bacterial β-lactamases. The penicillins (left) are the most important antibiotics*; the cephalosporins (right) having few specific indications. The β-lactam antibiotics are **bactericidal**. They produce their antimicrobial action by preventing the cross-linkage between the linear peptidoglycan polymer chains that make up the cell wall, e.g. by a pentaglycine bridge (●). This action is because a part of their structure (▬) resembles the D-alanyl-D-alanine of the peptide chains of the bacterial cell wall.

Benzylpenicillin was the first of the penicillins and remains important, but it is largely destroyed by gastric acid and must be given by injection. **Phenoxymethylpenicillin** has a similar antimicrobial spectrum, but is active orally. Many bacteria (including most staphylococci) are resistant to benzylpenicillin because they produce enzymes (β-lactamases, penicillinase) which open the β-lactam ring. The genetic control of β-lactamases often resides in transmissible plasmids (Chapter 35). Some penicillins e.g. **flucloxacillin** are effective against β-lactamase-producing staphylococci. Gram-negative, but not Gram-positive, bacteria possess an outer phospholipid membrane that may confer penicillin resistance by hindering access of the drugs to the cell wall. The **broad-spectrum** penicillins, such as **amoxycillin** and **ampicillin**, are more hydrophilic than benzylpenicillin and are active against some Gram-negative bacteria because they can pass through pores in the outer phospholipid membrane. Penicillinase-producing organisms are resistant to amoxycillin and ampicillin. The **antipseudomonal penicillins** (bottom left) are used mainly for the treatment of serious infections caused by *Pseudomonas aeruginosa***.

* Antibiotics are chemotherapeutic agents made by living micro-organisms rather than by chemical synthesis.
** *Pseudomonas aeruginosa* is a Gram-negative bacilli resistant to many antibiotics. It can cause serious opportunistic infections including pneumonia and septicaemia.

Penicillins have a very low toxicity, but high concentrations (renal failure, intrathecal administration) may produce encephalopathy, which can be fatal. **Hypersensitivity** is the most important side-effect of the penicillins which may cause rashes and, rarely, **anaphylactic reactions** which are fatal in about 10% of cases.

PENICILLINS

Benzylpenicillin remains one of the most useful antibiotics but it has a 'narrow spectrum' of activity, mainly against Gram-positive organisms. Benzylpenicillin is effective for treating pneumococcal, streptococcal, meningococcal and leptospiral infections. It is also valuable for the prophylaxis of clostridial gas gangrene. Most *Staphylococcus aureus*† now produces penicillinase. Benzylpenicillin is acid-labile and is therefore poorly absorbed orally. It is given by intramuscular injection, but large doses are painful and are given intravenously. Penicillin diffuses widely though the body tissues, but penetration into the brain is poor except when the meninges are inflamed. After intramuscular injection, peak plasma levels occur after 15–30 minutes and the drug is rapidly excreted (largely unchanged) by the kidneys. The elimination half-life, $t_{\frac{1}{2}}$, is normally 30 minutes, but is prolonged to about 10 hours in anuria. The renal tubular secretion of penicillin can be inhibited by organic acids such as **probenecid** and this results in higher and more prolonged plasma concentrations.

Procaine penicillin and **benethamine penicillin** are sparingly soluble salts of benzylpenicillin which are given by intramuscular injection. They have a prolonged action and procaine penicillin can be used when a rapid effect and high blood levels are unnecessary (e.g. syphilis and yaws). Benethamine penicillin is given only as a mixture with benzylpenicillin and procaine penicillin (Triplopen) usually as a 'starter' injection for a course of penicillin treatment.

Phenoxymethylpenicillin has the same spectrum as benzylpenicillin, but is less active. It is acid-stable and is given orally. However, its absorption is variable and it is only useful for very sensitive organisms, where a rapid action is unnecessary (streptococcal tonsillitis). Phenoxymethylpenicillin is useful in the prophylaxis of rheumatic fever.

Penicillinase-resistant penicillins—flucloxacillin. Flucloxacillin is indicated in infections due to penicillinase-producing penicillin-resistant staphylococci. It is a semisynthetic penicillin and is resistant to penicillinase because an isoxazolyl group at R_1 sterically hinders access of the enzyme to the β-lactam ring. Flucloxacillin is less effective than benzylpenicillin and should only be used in infections due to penicillinase-producing staphylococci (which includes about 90% of hospital-acquired staphylococcal infections). Flucloxacillin is well absorbed orally, but in severe infections it should be given by injection and not be used alone. Epidemic strains of *Staphylococcus aureus* resistant to methicillin (MRSA), flucloxacillin and other antibiotics are an increasing problem, especially in hospitals. Such infections are best treated with intravenous vancomycin.

Broad-spectrum penicillins. Ampicillin and **amoxycillin** are active against non-β-lactamase-producing Gram-positive bacteria, and because they diffuse into Gram-negative bacteria more readily than benzylpenicillin, they are also active against many strains of *Escherichia coli*, *Haemophilus influenzae* and *Salmonella*. For oral administration, amoxycillin is the drug of choice, because it is better absorbed than ampicillin which should be given parentally. Amoxycillin and ampicillin are inactivated by penicillinase-producing bacteria. Organisms that are resistant to amoxycillin include most *Staphylococcus aureus*, up to one-third of *Escherichia coli* strains and up to 10% of *Haemophilus influenzae* strains. Many bacterial β-lactamases are inhibited by **clavulanic acid**, and a mixture of this inhibitor with **amoxycillin (Augmentin)**, results in the antibiotic being effective against penicillinase-producing organisms. Augmentin is indicated in respiratory and urinary tract infections, which are confirmed resistant to amoxycillin.

Antipseudomonal penicillins. Piperacillin, **azlocillin** and **ticarcillin** are given by injection for serious infections with Gram-negative bacteria, especially *Pseudomonas aeruginosa*. They can be combined with aminoglycosides for the initial treatment of serious infection (e.g. septicaemia, endocarditis) when the bacterial cause has not been identified.

CEPHALOSPORINS

The cephalosporin antibiotics are widely used in most parts of the world, and increasingly in the United Kingdom. However, most must be given by injection, and there are very few indications when cephalosporins are indicated as the drug of first choice. The cephalosporins have the same mechanism of action as and similar pharmacology to penicillin. They may produce allergic reactions and cross-sensitivity to penicillin may occur. They are excreted mainly by the kidneys and their actions can be prolonged with probenecid. They all have a similar broad spectrum of antibacterial activity, although individual drugs have different activity against certain bacteria. **Cefadroxil** is administered orally and it is useful in urinary tract infections. **Cefuroxime** and **cephazolin** are given by injection often as a prophylactic in surgery (usually with metronidazole to provide cover against anaerobes). Cefuroxime is resistant to inactivation by bacterial β-lactamases and is used in serious infections when other antibiotics are ineffective. **Ceftazidime** has an increased range of activity against Gram-negative bacteria including *Pseudomonas aeruginosa*, but is less active than cefuroxime against Gram-positive organisms (e.g. *Staphylococcus aureus*). It reaches the central nervous system and may be the drug of choice in meningitis due to Gram-negative organisms in neonates.

VANCOMYCIN

Vancomycin is a bactericidal antibiotic that is not absorbed orally. It acts by inhibiting peptidoglycan formation and is active against many Gram-positive organisms. Intravenous vancomycin is being used increasingly in the treatment of patients with septicaemia or endocarditis due to methicillin-resistant strains of *Staphylococcus aureus*. It is the drug of choice (given orally) for antibiotic-associated pseudomembranous colitis (a serious complication of antibiotic therapy caused by a superinfection of the bowel by *Clostridium difficile*, which produces a toxin that damages the colonic mucosa). Rarely, vancomycin may cause renal failure or hearing loss.

† *Staphylococcus aureas* is a Gram-positive cocci. It is a common cause of infections including boils, wound infections, pneumonia, endocarditis and septicaemia.

37 Antimicrobial drugs that inhibit protein synthesis: aminoglycosides, tetracyclines, chloramphenicol and erythromycin

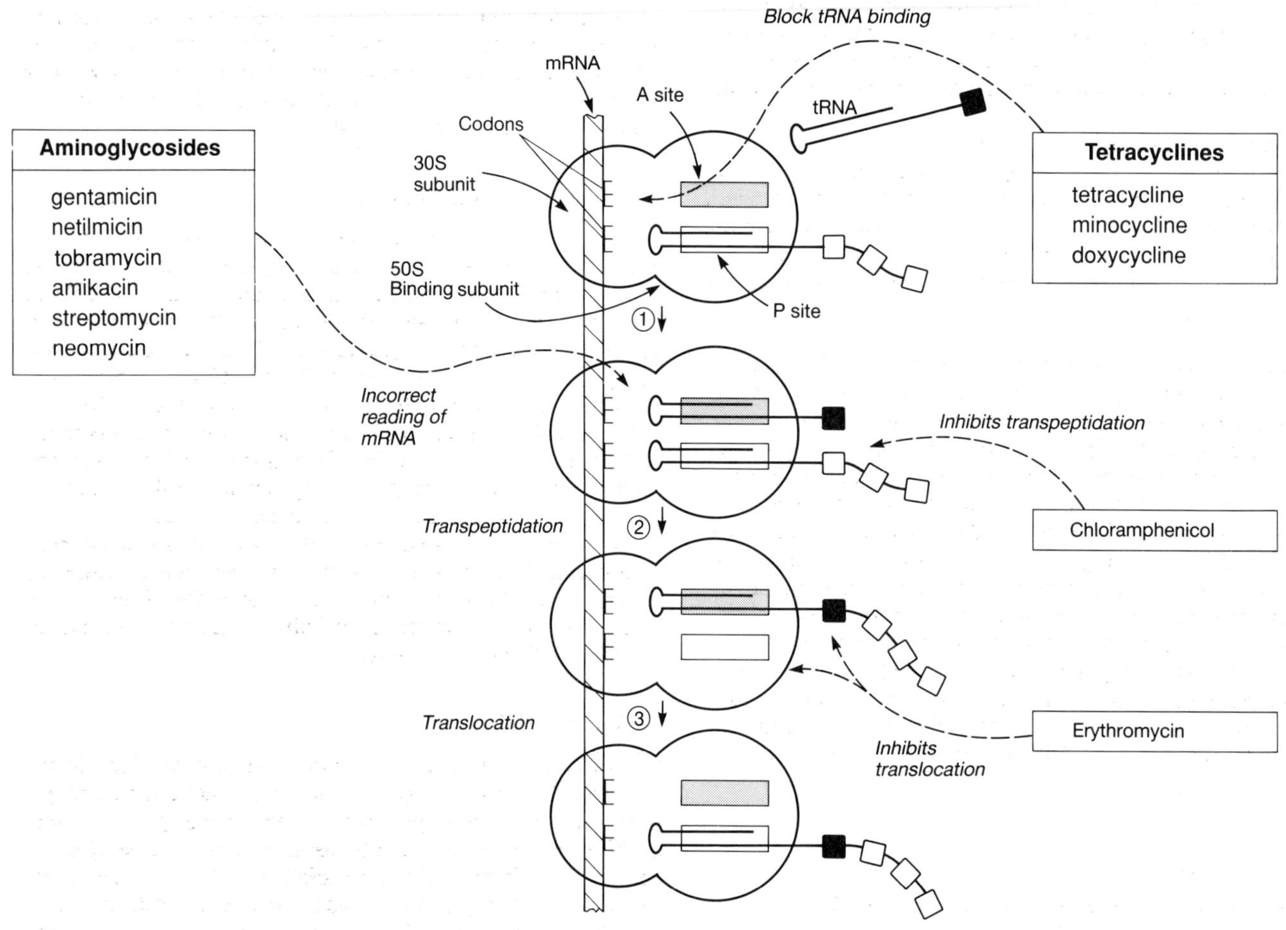

This group of antibiotics act by inhibiting bacterial protein synthesis. They are selectively toxic because bacterial ribosomes (the sites of protein synthesis) consist of a 50S and a 30S subunit, whilst mammalian ribosomes have a 60S and 40S subunit.

Proteins are built from amino acids, on ribosomes ( ), which move along (1–2–3) strands of messenger RNA (mRNA,) so that successive codons ( ) pass through an acceptor (aminoacyl, A site) for specific transfer RNA (tRNA) molecules which bear the next amino acid (top right ■) required to elongate the peptide chain. The **tetracyclines** (top right) and **aminoglycosides** (left) bind to the 30S subunit and *inhibit binding* of the aminoacyl-tRNA. In addition, the aminoglycosides cause *misreading* of mRNA, so that non-functional proteins are synthesized. The next step in peptide synthesis is transpeptidation (2), where the growing peptide chain (□) attached to the P (peptidyl,) site, is transferred to the amino acid (■) attached to the aminoacyl-tRNA at the A site. **Chloramphenicol** (middle right) *inhibits peptidyl transferase* activity of the 50S ribosomal subunit. Following transpeptidation, the peptide chain is translocated from site A to P (3) so that the A site is ready to accept the next aminoacyl-tRNA. **Erythromycin** (bottom right) binds to the 50S subunit and *inhibits translocation.*

The aminoglycosides such as **gentamicin** must be given by injection. They are valuable drugs in the treatment of severe infections, but are likely to produce nephrotoxic and ototoxic effects. The **tetracyclines** are orally active, wide-spectrum antibiotics, but increasing bacterial resistance has reduced their usefulness. **Erythromycin** has a similar antibacterial spectrum to benzylpenicillin and is a useful substitute in penicillin-sensitive patients. **Chloramphenicol** is effective against a wide range of organisms, but serious side-effects (e.g. aplastic anaemia) restrict its use.

AMINOGLYCOSIDES

The **aminoglycosides** are not absorbed orally and must be given by injection. They are bactericidal but have a narrow therapeutic index and are all potentially toxic. They are excreted by the kidney, and renal impairment results in accumulation and a greater risk of toxic side-effects. The most important side-effects of the aminoglycosides are damage to the VIIIth cranial nerve (**ototoxicity**) and damage to the **kidney**. These effects are dose related, and assays of blood aminoglycoside levels should be carried out regularly on all patients receiving aminoglycosides. Aminoglycosides may impair neuromuscular transmission and are, therefore, contraindicated in patients with myasthenia gravis.

Resistance to aminoglycosides arises from several mechanisms, the most important being the production of enzymes (plasmid controlled) that inactivate the drug by acetylation, phosphorylation or adenylylation. Other mechanisms are the alterations of the envelope to prevent drug access and alteration of the binding site on the 30S subunit so that the drug does not bind (streptomycin only).

Gentamicin is the most important aminoglycoside, its main use being in the 'empirical' treatment of acute life-threatening Gram-negative infections (e.g. *Pseudomonas aeruginosa*) in hospitals, until antibiotic sensitivities are known. Gentamicin may have a synergistic antimicrobial action with penicillin and vancomycin, and combinations with one of these agents are used in the treatment of streptococcal endocarditis. **Amikacin** is less affected by aminoglycoside-inactivating enzymes and is used in serious Gram-negative infections which are gentamicin resistant. **Netilmicin** is claimed to be less toxic than gentamicin. **Streptomycin** is active against *Mycobacterium tuberculosis* and its use is restricted to patients with tuberculosis. It has been largely replaced by rifampicin in combination with other drugs (e.g. isoniazid, pyrazinamide, ethambutol). Streptomycin causes dose-related **ototoxicity**, especially with prolonged or intensive therapy.

TETRACYCLINES

Tetracyclines are usually given orally but may be given by injection. Absorption from the gut is variable and is reduced by calcium ions (milk), magnesium ions (e.g. antacids) food and iron preparations. Tetracyclines are broad-spectrum antibiotics, but there are more suitable agents for most infections. However, they are the drug of choice for treating some infections due to intracellular organisms, because they penetrate macrophages well, e.g. *Chlamydia* (non-specific urethritis, trachoma, psittacosis) and rickettsia (Q-fever). Organisms sensitive to tetracyclines accumulate the drug partly by passive diffusion and partly by active transport. Resistant organisms do not accumulate the antibiotic and selection of microbial populations following the widespread use of tetracyclines in the past has resulted in many resistant strains of streptococci, staphylococci, pneumococci and coliforms. The genes for tetracycline resistance are transmitted by plasmids and are closely associated with those for other drugs to which the organisms will also be resistant (i.e. sulphonamides, aminoglycosides, chloramphenicol). Tetracyclines cause discoloration of teeth in the young and should be avoided in children up to 8 years of age and in pregnant or lactating women. Diarrhoea and nausea may occur. Overgrowth with *Candida albicans* in the mouth or bowel sometimes leads to thrush.

CHLORAMPHENICOL

Chloramphenicol is given orally or by intravenous injection. It is effective against a wide range of organisms. Unfortunately, serious side-effects, which include bone marrow aplasia (incidence about 1 in 40 000—usually fatal), reversible (dose-related) suppression of red and white blood cells, encephalopathy and optic neuritis, restrict its use. Chloramphenicol is indicated in typhoid fever and *Haemophilus influenzae* meningitis. It is metabolized mainly in the liver and penetrates widely, including the brain. Chloramphenicol inhibits the metabolism of other drugs and may potentiate the actions of phenytoin, sulphonylureas and oral anticoagulants. Periodic blood counts are required, especially when the drug is given in high doses, for a long time, to patients with renal failure, or to neonates. The latter cannot metabolize the drug rapidly and accumulation causes 'grey baby' syndrome, i.e. pallor, abdominal distension, vomiting and collapse.

ERYTHROMYCIN

Erythromycin is usually given orally but can be given intravenously. It has a similar antimicrobial spectrum to benzylpenicillin (i.e. narrow spectrum, mainly active against Gram-positive organisms) and can be used as an alternative drug in penicillin-sensitive patients, especially in infections caused by streptococci, staphylococci, pneumococci and clostridia. It is specifically indicated in *Mycoplasma* pneumonia and Legionnaires' disease. Erythromycin is metabolized by the liver and dosage reduction in renal failure is unnecessary unless severe. The estolate may cause liver damage and should not be used. Erythromycin in high doses may cause nausea and vomiting. Resistance to erythromycin may occur due to plasmid-controlled alteration of its receptor on the 50S subunit of the bacterial ribosomes.

38 Antifungal and antiviral drugs

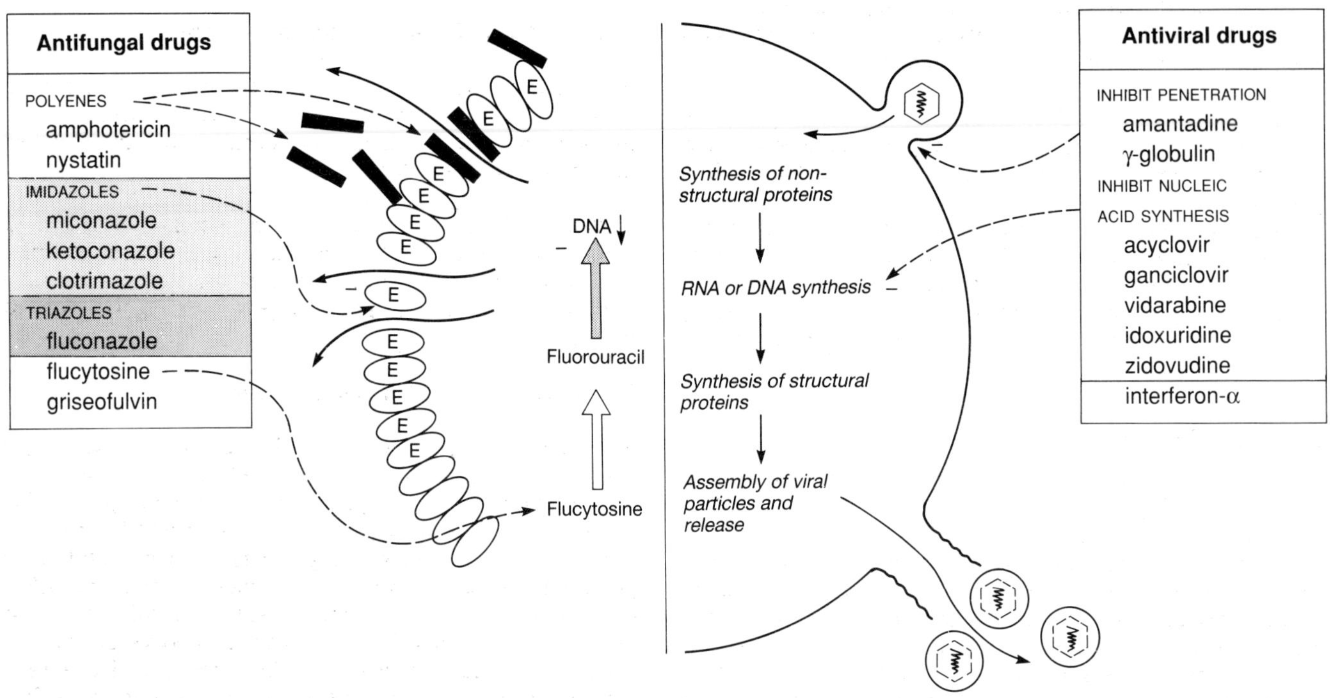

Fungal infections (mycoses) may be superficial or systemic, the latter occurring mostly in immunocompromised patients (AIDS patients, corticosteroids, anticancer drugs). There are not many effective antifungal drugs (left) and the first-line drug in systemic mycoses, **amphotericin**, is highly toxic. Amphotericin is a polyene antibiotic that interacts (left, ▬) with ergosterol (E) in the fungal cell membrane and forms pores through which essential fungal cell constituents are lost (←). The drug is selectively toxic because in human cells the major sterol is cholesterol rather than ergosterol. **Flucytosine** (bottom left) is much less toxic than amphotericin, but its use is limited because it has a narrow spectrum and resistance can develop rapidly during therapy. Flucytosine is converted in fungal cells, but not in human cells, into fluorouracil (⇨) which inhibits DNA synthesis (Chapter 40). The **imidazoles** (left, □), which are widely used topically, are broad-spectrum antifungal drugs that act by inhibiting ergosterol synthesis. The **triazoles** (left, □) are newer drugs, structurally similar to the imidazoles but with a wider range of antifungal activity. **Griseofulvin** is given orally and is useful for some dermatophyte infections, particularly chronic nail infections. Treatment may need to be prolonged for months. The mechanism of action of griseofulvin may involve interference with microtubule function.

Viruses are intracellular parasites that lack independent metabolism and can replicate only within living host cells. Since their replication cycle is so intimately connected with the metabolic processes of the host cell, it has proved extremely difficult to produce drugs that are selectively toxic to viruses. For this reason, vaccines have been the main method for controlling viral infections (e.g. poliomyelitis, rabies, yellow fever, measles, mumps, rubella). Some effective antiviral drugs (right) have been produced and although they are of limited use, they have transformed the treatment of several diseases, notably those caused by Herpes virus infections. Viral replication involves several steps (right figure). **Amantadine** and **γ-globulin** (top right) inhibit penetration of the cell by the virus ( ) but most antiviral drugs (bottom right) are **nucleoside analogues** that interfere with viral (and often human) nucleic acid synthesis. Newer drugs, especially **acyclovir** which is the most useful agent, are more selectively antiviral, because they are inactive until phosphorylated by enzymes that are preferentially synthesized by the virus. **Interferon-α** is an antiviral protein that is normally produced by leucocytes, but can now be obtained by recombinant DNA technology. It is given by intramuscular injection in the treatment of chronic persistent hepatitis (both B and non-A, non-B).

FUNGAL INFECTIONS

There are three main groups of fungi that cause disease in man.

1 **Moulds** (filamentous fungi) grow as long filaments which intertwine to form a mycelium. Examples are the *dermatophytes*, so called because of their ability to digest keratin, which cause infections of the skin, nails and hair, and *Aspergillus fumigatus* which may cause pulmonary or disseminated aspergillosis.

2 **True yeasts** are unicellular round or oval fungi, e.g. *Cryptococcus neoformans* which may cause cryptococcal meningitis or pulmonary infections, usually only in immunocompromised patients.

3 **Yeast-like fungi** are similar to yeasts but may also form long non-branching filaments. An important example is *Candida albicans*, which is a common commensal organism in the gut, mouth and vagina. It causes a wide range of disease including oral thrush, vaginitis, endocarditis and septicaemia (often fatal).

POLYENES

Amphotericin is a wide-spectrum antifungal drug used to treat potentially fatal systemic infections due to aspergillus, candida or cryptococcus. It is poorly absorbed orally and is given by intravenous infusion, or intrathecally, when the central nervous system is involved. Adverse effects are very common and most patients develop fever, chills and nausea. Long-term therapy almost inevitably causes renal damage, which is reversible only if detected early. **Nystatin** is too toxic for parenteral use. It is mainly used for *Candida albicans* infections of the skin (cream or ointment) and mucous membranes (tablets sucked in the mouth, vaginal pessaries). Oropharyngeal candidiasis (thrush) is one of the most common features of AIDS and is sometimes a sequel to the use of broad-spectrum antibiotics, anticancer drugs or corticosteroids.

FLUCYTOSINE

Flucytosine is given orally or by intravenous infusion. It is only active against yeasts and is used mainly to treat systemic candidiasis or cryptococcal infections. As resistance often develops rapidly, flucytosine may be given in combination with amphotericin. The drugs act synergistically and the combination is effective in cryptococcal meningitis.

IMIDAZOLES

Imidazoles are wide-spectrum antifungal drugs to which resistance rarely develops. Except for ketoconazole the imidazoles are poorly absorbed orally. **Clotrimazole**, **econazole** and **miconazole** are widely used topically in the treatment of dermatophyte and *Candida albicans* infections. **Miconazole** is used intravenously in systemic infections in patients who cannot tolerate amphotericin. It may cause nausea and vomiting, faintness and anaphylaxis. **Ketoconazole** is well absorbed orally, and has been used in the treatment of local and systemic mycoses. Enthusiasm for ketoconazole has declined because it may cause hepatic necrosis and adrenal suppression.

TRIAZOLES

Fluconazole may be given orally or intravenously and has been successfully used in a wide range of superficial and systemic mycoses (not *Aspergillus*). Unlike ketoconazole, it is not hepatotoxic and does not inhibit steroid synthesis. **Itraconazole** is absorbed orally and unlike the imidazoles and fluconazole, it is active against *Aspergillus*.

ANTIVIRAL DRUGS

Drugs that stop the virus entering the host cells

Amantadine is given orally and has been used rather unenthusiastically for the prophylaxis of influenza A infections. The major drawbacks are its narrow spectrum and the fact that influenza vaccine is often preferable.

γ-Globulin. Human immunoglobulin contains specific antibodies against superficial antigens of viruses and can interfere with their entry into the host cells. Normal immunoglobulin injections are used to give temporary protection against hepatitis A.

Drugs that inhibit nucleic acid synthesis

Acyclovir (acycloguanosine). The herpes viruses e.g. *Herpes simplex* (HSV) and *Varicella zoster* (VZV) contain a thymidine kinase which converts acyclovir to a monophosphate. The monophosphate is subsequently phosphorylated by host cell enzymes to acycloguanosine triphosphate which inhibits viral DNA polymerase and viral DNA synthesis. Acyclovir is selectively toxic because the thymidine kinase of uninfected host cells activates only a little of the drug and the DNA polymerase of herpes virus has a much higher affinity for the activated drug than the cellular DNA polymerase. Acyclovir is active against Herpes viruses but does not eradicate them. It is effective topically, orally and parenterally and the appropriate route depends on the site and severity of the infection. Acyclovir is widely used in the treatment of HSV genital infections and high oral doses are effective in severe shingles, a painful condition caused by reactivation of a previous infection with VZV (i.e. chickenpox). **Idoxuridine** is also active against HSV but it is too toxic except for topical use in severe herpetic infections of the skin, eye and external genitalia. Other drugs have largely superseded idoxuridine.

Ganciclovir must be given intravenously and, because of its toxicity (neutropenia), it is used only to treat severe cytomegalovirus (CMV) infections in immunocompromised patients. Cytomegalovirus is resistant to acyclovir because it does not code for thymidine kinase.

Vidarabine (adenine arabinoside) is converted to the triphosphate in the host cells and inhibits viral DNA polymerase much more than host cell polymerase. Vidarabine is used (by slow intravenous infusion) in immunosuppressed patients to treat serious infections caused by Herpes viruses. Vidarabine is relatively non-toxic but may cause mild bone marrow depression.

Zidovudine (3-azido-3-deoxythymidine) inhibits human immunodeficiency virus (HIV) and is used orally in the treatment of acquired immunodeficiency syndrome (AIDS). The drug is activated by triple phosphorylation and then binds to reverse transcriptase for which it has 100 times the affinity than it has for cellular DNA polymerases. The drug is incorporated into the DNA chain and reverse transcription comes to a halt. Resistance develops over 12–18 months and some patients cannot tolerate the severe side-effects which include anaemia, neutropenia, nausea, insomnia, headaches and myalgia.

39 Antiprotozoal drugs

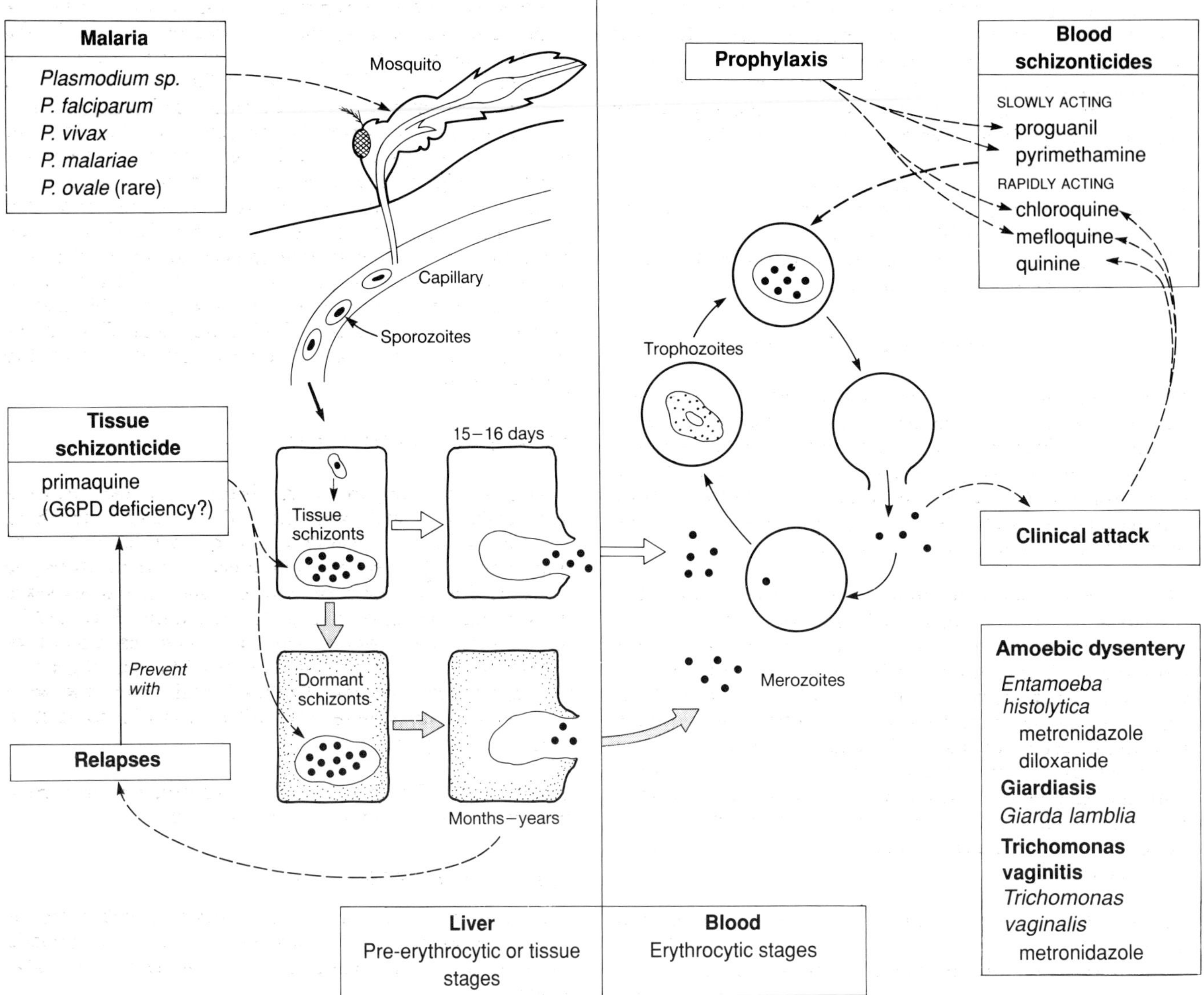

Protozoal infections cause bowel disease (amoebic dysentery, giardiasis), vaginitis (bottom right) and malaria (top left). Malaria is the most serious of these, and although it is not endemic in Europe or North America, travellers to malarial areas risk infection. This risk can be greatly reduced by taking prophylactic drugs (prophylaxis, top right) but drug-resistant malaria is an increasing problem in many parts of the world. There is no prophylactic drug treatment for other protozoal infections.

Malaria is caused by four species of protozoa (top left) that have part of their life cycle in the female *Anopheles* mosquito. When a mosquito bites a human it injects sporozoites into a capillary (⊙, top left) and these are carried in the blood to the liver where they multiply and form tissue schizonts. This is the pre-erythrocytic or primary tissue stage of the disease (left figure). After 5–16 days the schizonts rupture and release (⇨) thousands of merozoites (●) which infect red blood cells (○) and start the erythrocytic stage of the disease (right figure). In the case of *P. vivax* and *P. ovale* (but not *P. falciparum*) some of the schizonts in the liver remain dormant (▒) and these may rupture months or years later, causing a relapse of the disease (⇨).

Most antimalarials are toxic to the erythrocytic schizonts (blood schizonticides, top right) and the rapidly acting ones (**chloroquine**, **quinine**, **mefloquine**) are used to treat clinical attacks of malaria. **Pyrimethamine** and **proguanil** act too slowly for this purpose and they are used to provide prophylaxis, especially in areas where the parasite is resistant to chloroquine. Chloroquine and mefloquine are used for both prophylaxis and treatment (quinine is too toxic). **Primaquine** (left) is a tissue schizonticide used to eliminate the schizonts in the liver (radical cure) once the clinical attack is controlled with chloroquine or quinine.

Infections with other protozoa (bottom right) are treated mainly with **metronidazole**.

MALARIA

Clinical attacks are characterized by paroxysms of fever that coincide with the release of erythrocytic schizonts at the end of each schizogonic cycle. In *P. vivax* infections (the most common in humans) there is a 48-hour cycle (i.e. fever on day 1 and 3) and the disease is called benign tertian malaria. Malignant tertian malaria is due to infection with *P. falciparum*. It is the most dangerous form of the disease and the only type of acute malaria that is likely to cause death in previously healthy persons (usually due to cerebral or renal complications).

Relapses. In the case of *P. vivax* and *P. ovale* infections, some schizonts may remain in the liver for months or years before being released into the blood and causing a relapse of the disease. Only **primaquine** can kill the liver schizonts and so produce a radical cure in these infections.

BLOOD SCHIZONTICIDES (rapidly acting)

Chloroquine usually controls the fever of most forms of malaria within 24–48 hours. It has two disadvantages: (1) it has no action on the liver schizonts and therefore cannot produce a radical cure in *vivax* and *ovale* infections; and (2) in most areas of the world, *P. falciparum* has become resistant to the drug. Chloroquine is usually given orally but may be given by intravenous infusion to seriously ill patients.

Mechanism of action. Chloroquine is concentrated 100-fold in parasitized erythrocytes compared with normal erythrocytes, because degradation of haemoglobin by *Plasmodia* releases ferriprotoporphyrin IX, which acts as a chloroquine receptor. It is not known how the chloroquine concentrated in the erythrocytes kills the malarial parasite, but possible mechanisms involve intercalation (Chapter 40) and changes in plasmodial lysosomal pH. Malarial parasites exposed to sublethal concentrations of chloroquine eventually become resistant to the drug. At this stage, little chloroquine can be found in the parasite, suggesting that resistance is due to failure of the drug to penetrate the cell wall.

Adverse effects. These are unusual with the low doses used for prophylaxis. The higher doses used for treatment may cause nausea, vomiting, diarrhoea, rashes, pruritis and, rarely, psychoses. Prolonged administration of high doses may irreversibly damage the retina.

Quinine and **mefloquine** are used orally to treat *P. falciparum* infections (malignant tertian malaria) resistant to chloroquine. Quinine can be given by intravenous infusion if necessary (e.g. unconsciousness). A 7-day course of quinine is followed by Fansidar (see later) or given with tetracycline (if Fansidar resistant). Combined therapy is not necessary with mefloquine which is more potent and less toxic than quinine.

Adverse effects of quinine include abdominal pain, nausea, tinnitus, headache, blindness, hypersensitivity reactions, haemolysis and, rarely, leucopenia, agranulocytosis and thrombocytopenic purpura. Overdoses cause profound hypotension due to peripheral vasodilation and myocardial depression (see quinidine, Chapter 17). The mechanism of action of quinine and mefloquine is unknown.

BLOOD SCHIZONTICIDES (slowly acting)

Pyrimethamine *and* **proguanil** are effective schizonticides, but their action is too slow to treat acute attacks.

Mechanism of action. Pyrimethamine and the active metabolite of proguanil (cycloguanil) are folate antagonists. They inhibit dihydrofolate reductase and, by preventing the regeneration of tetrahydrofolate, they inhibit DNA synthesis and cell division. The drugs are selectively toxic because they have 1000 times the affinity for the plasmodial enzyme than they have the human enzyme (compare with methotrexate, Chapter 40, which has a high affinity for the human enzyme). In areas where *P. falciparum* is resistant to choloroquine, pyrimethamine is given in combination with a sulphonamide (Fansidar) or sulphone (Maloprim). The latter drugs (sulfadoxine and dapsone, respectively) act on the same pathway as pyrimethamine, but at a different point (Chapter 35), and this sequential blockade is more effective than the action of either drug alone. Chloroquine is given concurrently because *P. vivax* is now often resistant to pyrimethamine.

TISSUE SCHIZONTICIDE

Primaquine is an important drug because it is the only antimalarial that will kill the schizonts of *P. vivax* and *P. ovale* lying dormant in the liver. However, it is of no value in treating clinical attacks because it has little effect on the erythrocytic schizonts. The mechanism of action of primaquine is unknown. It seems that oxidative damage to the parasite is caused by active metabolites, which may also cause haemolysis of erythrocytes in persons with an inherited deficiency of glucose-6-phosphate dehydrogenase (G6PD). For this reason, the blood of patients should be tested for G6PD activity before starting treatment with primaquine.

Adverse effects of primaquine include nausea, vomiting, bone marrow depression and haemolytic anaemia.

AMOEBIC DYSENTERY

This is caused by infection with *Entamoeba histolytica*. Metronidazole is used in acute infections, but in asymptomatic infections, where cysts are present, diloxanide furoate is also necessary.

GIARDIASIS

Giardia lamblia is a flagellate pear-shaped protozoan. It is a common bowel pathogen causing flatulence and diarrhoea. Metronidazole is effective.

TRICHOMONAS VAGINITIS

Trichomonas vaginalis is a common cause of vaginal discharge and occasionally causes urethritis in both sexes. Metronidazole is usually very effective.

Metronidazole, in addition to its antiprotozoal action, also has high activity against anaerobic bacteria (e.g. *Bacteroides fragilis*). The drug is reduced to active metabolites which interfere with nucleic acid function. It can be given intravenously in severe sepsis. Adverse effects are infrequent.

40 Drugs used in cancer

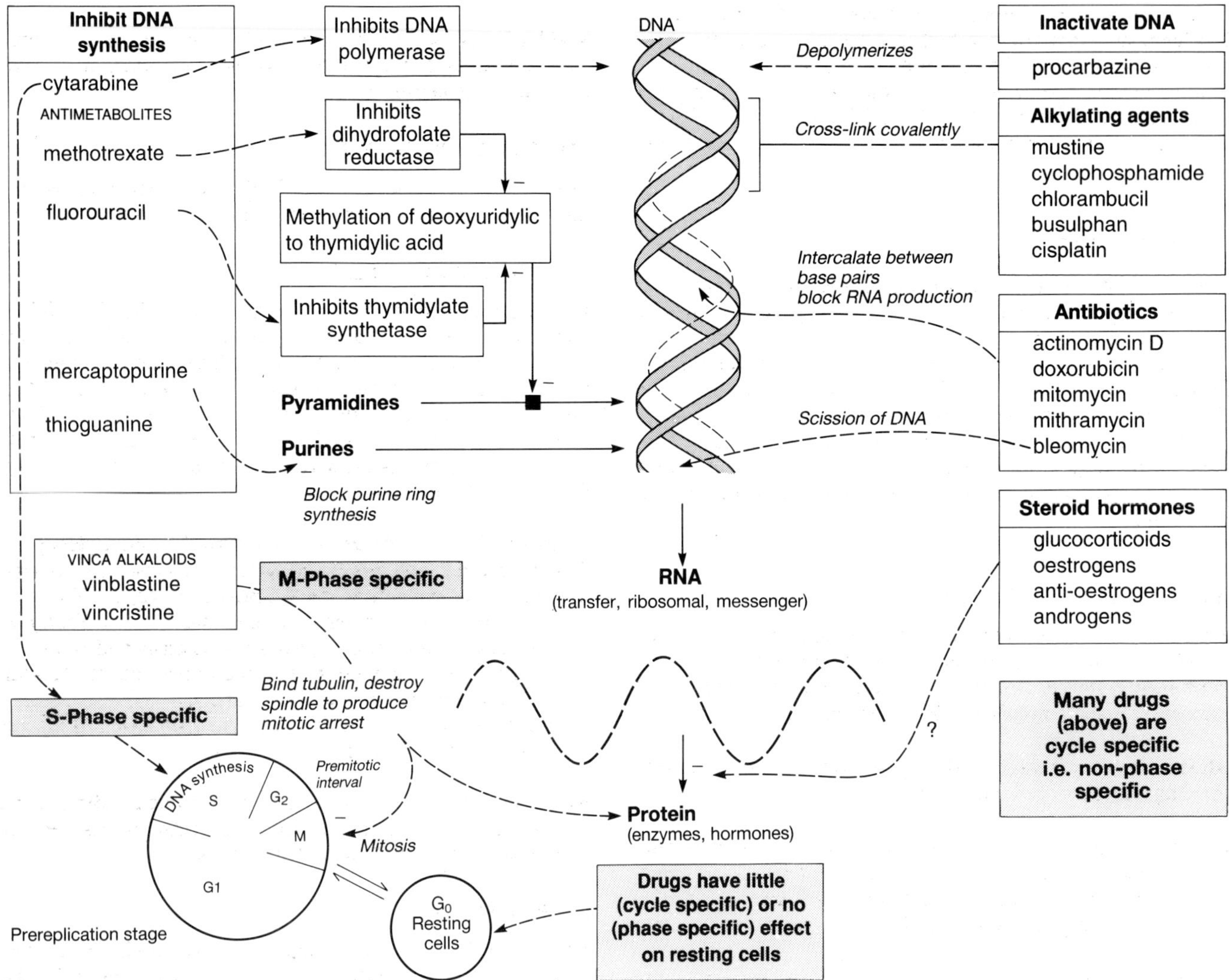

The aim of treatment in patients with cancer is cure, or if this is not possible, effective palliation. Many cancers present as localized tumour masses, but surgery or radiotherapy often fail to eradicate the disease, which eventually becomes widespread. For this reason, there is a trend to incorporate systemic treatment with local treatment at the time of diagnosis.

Drugs used to treat cancer inhibit the mechanisms of cell proliferation. They are, therefore, toxic to both tumour cells and proliferating normal cells, especially in the *bone marrow*, *gastrointestinal epithelium* and *hair follicles*. The **selectivity** of cytotoxic drugs occurs because in malignant tumours a higher proportion of the component cells are undergoing division than in normal proliferating tissues.

Anticancer drugs are classified according to their sites of action along the synthetic pathway of cellular macromolecules (top). Some drugs are only effective during part of the cell cycle (**phase-specific drugs**, left), whilst others (**cycle-specific drugs**, right) are cytotoxic throughout the cell cycle (lower figure).

Alkylating agents (top right) readily form covalent bonds. They react with the bases in DNA and prevent cell division by cross-linking the two strands of the double helix. Several **antibiotics** (middle right) isolated from various species of *Streptomyces* also interact with DNA and are widely used as anticancer drugs. Some cytotoxic drugs act by interfering with DNA synthesis (top left). These agents are **antimetabolites** and inhibit purine or pyrimidine synthesis. One is a folic acid antagonist (methotrexate). The **vinca alkaloids** (bottom left) inhibit mitosis by binding to the microtubular proteins necessary for spindle formation. A miscellaneous group of drugs is also used in the treatment of cancer, e.g. procarbazine. **Steroid hormones** and hormone antagonists (lower right) are often used in the treatment of cancer. **Combinations** of cytotoxic drugs may be strikingly more successful than single drugs in the treatment of some cancers (e.g. Hodgkin's disease).

The administration of cytotoxic drugs may be associated with unpleasant and even life-threatening **adverse effects**. Individual drugs sometimes have specific toxic effects, but general adverse effects common to many agents include nausea and vomiting (reduced by antiemetics such as prochlorperazine, dexamethasone and ondansetron), oral and intestinal ulceration, diarrhoea, alopecia and bone marrow suppression, which can decrease production of any or all the formed elements of blood. Leucopenia is associated with an increased risk of opportunistic infections; thrombocytopenia leads to bleeding, and decreased red cell formation causes anaemia. *Vincristine* and *bleomycin* are exceptions that do not cause myelosuppression.

DRUG COMBINATIONS

The administration of combinations of drugs given intermittently often produces better results than more continuous treatment with a single drug. The rationale is that a combination of drugs with different toxic effects and affecting different biochemical pathways has higher antitumour activity without additive toxicity. For example, combination of mustine, vincristine, procarbazine and prednisone (MOPP) induces remission in 80% of patients with Hodgkin's disease, whilst the drugs used individually induce remission in less than 40% of patients.

SELECTIVITY

The selectivity of antitumour drugs is marginal at best. Their beneficial effects depend on the bone marrow cells recovering faster than the tumour cells after drug administration. Following marrow recovery, further drug can be given, and because a fixed proportion of tumour cells are killed during each period of drug administration, the tumour may eventually be eradicated. In practice, the response of tumours to chemotherapy ranges from 'cure', e.g. acute lymphoblastic leukaemia in children, to being completely refractory, e.g. colorectal carcinoma, melanoma.

ALKYLATING AGENTS

These drugs are widely used in cancer chemotherapy. Prolonged usage often affects gametogenesis severely; most males become permanently sterile. The drugs are associated with an increased incidence of acute non-lymphocytic leukaemia.

Mustine is given intravenously in Hodgkin's disease. It is very toxic and causes severe vomiting.

Cyclophosphamide is metabolized in the liver forming several active metabolites. One metabolite, acrolein, occasionally causes haemorrhagic cystitis, a serious complication. Cyclophosphamide is extensively used in a wide variety of cancers.

Chlorambucil is given orally. It is tending to replace other alkylating agents because it has milder adverse effects.

CYTOTOXIC ANTIBIOTICS

Actinomycin D possesses a phenoxazone ring which slips between neighbouring base pairs in DNA. This *intercalation* process forces the base pairs apart and 'lengthens' the double helical DNA so it cannot be an effective template for RNA synthesis. Most other antibiotics used in the treatment of cancer are also *intercalating agents*, although mitomycin may be an alkylating agent and bleomycin causes single-strand breaks in RNA.

Bleomycin is unusual in that it spares the bone marrow, but it causes progressive pulmonary fibrosis in about 5% of patients.

Doxorubicin is one of the most successful antitumour drugs and is used in acute leukaemias, lymphomas and a variety of solid tumours. High cumulative doses are cardiotoxic, probably because oxygen free radicals are formed which are not inactivated in the heart as it lacks catalase.

VINCA ALKALOIDS

Vincristine is used in acute lymphoblastic leukaemia, lymphomas and some solid tumours. It has toxic effects on peripheral and autonomic nerves.

Vinblastine is used in the treatment of lymphomas and testicular teratomas. It causes more myelosuppression than vincristine but is less neurotoxic.

MISCELLANEOUS DRUGS

Procarbazine is a first-line agent in the treatment of Hodgkin's disease in combination with other drugs (MOPP).

ANTIMETABOLITES

Folic acid antagonists. *Methotrexate* competitively inhibits dihydrofolate reductase and prevents the regeneration of tetrahydrofolic acid and the co-enzyme, methylene tetrahydrofolate, which is essential for the conversion of deoxyuridylic acid to thymidylic acid. Since rapidly dividing cells require an abundant supply of deoxythymidylate for the synthesis of DNA, methotrexate prevents the division of cells. It is given in many forms of malignant disease.

Antipyrimidines. *Fluorouracil* is converted to fluorodeoxyuridylic acid which inhibits thymidylate synthetase, the enzyme responsible for converting deoxyuridylate to thymidylic acid. This impairs DNA synthesis by reducing the availability of thymidylic acid. It is mainly given intravenously and is used in the treatment of solid tumours, especially breast cancer. It is the drug of choice for metastatic colon cancer.

Cytarabine has an uncertain mechanism of action. It is used in myeloblastic leukaemia.

Antipurines impair the synthesis of purine nucleotides but the mechanisms involved are not clear. *Mercaptopurine* is used for maintenance therapy in acute leukaemias.

HORMONES

Glucocorticoids (e.g. *prednisolone*) inhibit cell division by interfering with DNA synthesis. They are widely used in the treatment of leukaemias, lymphomas and breast cancer.

Sex hormones and antagonists. The growth of some tumours is partly dependent upon hormones, especially carcinoma of the breast and prostate. Removal of the gland producing the hormone, the administration of hormones with the opposite action or the administration of an antagonist, may induce tumour regression. *Tamoxifen*, an oestrogen antagonist, is widely used in the treatment of postmenopausal metastatic breast cancer. In prostatic cancer, *stilboestrol* produces remission in 80% of cases. Unfortunately, the effects of hormones are usually temporary, because hormone-independent cells eventually predominate.

IMMUNOSUPPRESSANTS

These are used to prevent tissue rejection after organ transplantation and to treat autoimmune and collagen diseases.

Azathioprine is converted to mercaptopurine in the body and is widely used in combination with *prednisolone*. The glucocorticoids act mainly on polymorph and macrophage activity.

Cyclosporin is a potent immunosuppressant used especially to prevent rejection of organ and tissue transplants. It is not myelotoxic but may cause kidney damage.

Index